SHEKNOWS.com.

PRESENTS:

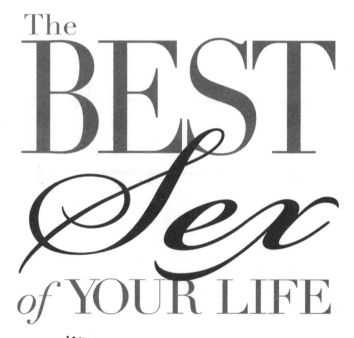

The
BEST
Sex
of YOUR LIFE

2010

JUL   W1

JUL 2010

SHEKNOWS.com.

PRESENTS:

The
BEST
Sex
of YOUR LIFE

101 Secrets
EVERY WOMAN
Should
KNOW

Jennifer Hunt
& Dan Baritchi

Authors of *1,001 Best Places to Have Sex in America*

Foreword by Nancy J. Price and Betsy Bailey,
founding editors, SheKnows.com

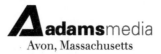

Aadamsmedia
Avon, Massachusetts

Published by
Adams Media, a division of F+W Media, Inc.
57 Littlefield Street, Avon, MA 02322. U.S.A.
www.adamsmedia.com

ISBN 10: 1-60550-143-3
ISBN 13: 978-1-60550-143-7

Printed in the United States of America.

10 9 8 7 6 5 4 3 2 1

Library of Congress Cataloging-in-Publication Data
is available from the publisher.

SheKnows.com Presents: The Best Sex of Your Life is intended as a reference volume only. In light of the complex, individual, and specific nature of health conditions, this book is not intended to replace professional medical advice. The ideas, procedures, and suggestions in this book are intended to supplement, not replace, the advice of a trained professional. Consult your physician before adopting the suggestions in this book, as well as about any condition that may require diagnosis or medical attention. The author, SheKnows.com, and publisher disclaim any liability arising directly or indirectly from the use of this book.

This publication is designed to provide accurate and authoritative information with regard to the subject matter covered. It is sold with the understanding that the publisher is not engaged in rendering legal, accounting, or other professional advice. If legal advice or other expert assistance is required, the services of a competent professional person should be sought.
—From a *Declaration of Principles* jointly adopted by a Committee of the American Bar Association and a Committee of Publishers and Associations

Many of the designations used by manufacturers and sellers to distinguish their product are claimed as trademarks. Where those designations appear in this book and Adams Media was aware of a trademark claim, the designations have been printed with initial capital letters.

This book is available at quantity discounts for bulk purchases.

For information, please call 1-800-289-0963.

Acknowledgments

So many people helped make this book a reality, and we would like to extend our profound and sincere gratitude to each of them.

The following people are key contributors to both AskDan AndJennifer.com and this book. Their knowledge, skills, and wisdom help us all.

Kaylen Shubrick, our amazing writer and editor who helps turn our thoughts and videos into words.

Paul Carlson (*www.PersonalChanges.com*), life coach and CCHt (Certified Clinical Hypnotherapist). His background provides him with a unique ability to provide guidance and coaching for those who want a better, happier, and more successful personal and business life.

Melody Brooke (*www.ThisIsGreatSex.com*), Professional and Marriage and Family Counselor, international speaker, author, and founder of ThisIsGreatSex.com.

The Beautiful Kind (*www.TheBeautifulKind.com*), kink expert, sex writer, and consultant, as well as a sex worker specializing in fetishes and surrogacy (a sexual surrogate is someone who helps others overcome social and sexual issues through hands-on intimacy).

In addition, we would like to thank the following people for making this book possible:

Neil Salkind (*www.studiob.com/salkindagency*), our amazing literary agent; and all of the amazing people at Adams Media (*www.adamsmedia.com*), our publisher, for their incredible help and support while writing this book.

And last, but not least, we extend our profound thanks to you for reading this book. We hope you have as much fun reading it as we did writing it!

Dedication

For Mom (1947–2009) Thank you Mom for your unconditional love, acceptance, and willingness to talk openly and honestly, even about the hard topics.

To Jennifer, my best friend, my lover, my partner in crime. Thank you for helping me find the light.

P.S. I love you.

Contents

Foreword   ix

Introduction   xi

Appendix A: Recommended Resources   181

Appendix B: The 101 Secrets Every Woman Should Know   193

Index   203

About the Authors   211

Foreword

Have you ever heard anyone say that, for men, everything revolves around sex? We all know it is a little more complicated than that—and, of course, there are always exceptions to the rule—but we also know there are good reasons sex is so important to men. As women, we are well served when we give our sexual needs and desires priority as well. Sex can be a salve for a bad day at work, an incredibly fun way to spend an evening (or morning, or afternoon), and a way to bring us closer to our partners. After all, don't you find that you are a much happier person and that your relationship is usually much smoother sailing when you and your man are both sexually satisfied?

An active, vital sex life is not only a key component in a strong relationship, it is healthy and empowering for women. When it comes right down to it, is there anyone stronger or more powerful than a confident woman who is secure in her sexuality?

Maybe you want to be that lusty, sexually confident partner, but you feel a little shy and inhibited. Maybe you have a lot more questions than answers. After all, even in our supposedly enlightened and liberated times, there are still lots of taboos when it comes to the sexy details of a satisfying romp. *Sex and the City* was a *huge* step in the right direction, but if you only have Hollywood as your primary source of information, there are still significant gaps in your sexual education. If so, pick a page—any page—of this book and be prepared to learn something. It is chock full of ideas for mixing it up, being creative and keeping your sex life fresh and interesting.

It's funny, because we didn't necessarily realize how many gaps we had in our education ten years ago when we honored the request of SheKnows.com community members and added a Sex Talk ("for her eyes only!") forum to the message boards.

What happened in this community was a revelation. Women not only wanted to talk about sex, they wanted to *learn more about it*, improve the experience, and try new things in bed (or out, as the case may be). Even more importantly, they had extremely valuable information to share. Never particularly prudish, it was still an eye-opener to see what women would talk about when freed from the constraints of a face-to-face conversation. We found ourselves saying, "My, my, my—we hadn't even considered *that*. What? Really? They make products like *that*? Huh?" Suddenly, there were whole new worlds to explore.

That's the point of this book: to be a refreshingly fun primer about how to have a better time in bed . . . or, really, a better time wherever the mood takes you. It's not intended to be a serious relationship tome at all, and yet you might find it has a better effect on your relationship than any other strategy you've ever tried.

It is our hope that as you read this book you get to know more about yourself and your needs and desires, and how to make a lot of memories that will warm you up—and make you smile—for years to come.

**Betsy Bailey and Nancy J. Price, Founders
and Executive Editors**
SheKnows.com

Introduction

How's your sex life? If your immediate answer is "Amazing," then feel free to put down this book. But, if your sex life could use a little tinkering here and there, or even a major overhaul, come closer. That's better. Throughout the course of this book, we will whisper 101 secrets in your ear that will put you well on your way to having amazing sex. Trust us, the next time you're getting it on, you'll be moaning so loudly that your upstairs neighbors will think their apartment is haunted.

Maybe you've never had sex. Or, maybe you already know how to have good sex . . . either way we want you to have the best sex of your life. We're talking about mind-blowing, off-the-charts, nails-down-the-back sex. Don't feel bad if you haven't been having it. When it comes to mastering everything, we all need a good teacher and practice. Think of us as your secret muse. We'll give you the dish on secrets your girlfriends won't even talk about. For starters, did you know it's possible for *all* women to experience multiple orgasms? We've got the lowdown on how. Want to know what men are thinking? We offer "He Says . . ." tips throughout that tell you what guys commonly want, think, and feel.

Though not everything we suggest will be something that you are comfortable with right away, you'll definitely discover some new tips and tricks and have your mind opened to new ideas to try in the bedroom that you may have never even considered. Within this book we'll share with you the one thing you need to know to improve your oral sex skills from good to great (it's not what you think!), teach you the best sex position for *your* pleasure, explain how to use household objects in kinky ways, and empower you to unleash your inner seductress so your man doesn't even stand a chance. But, of course, we don't stop there.

We will also tackle how to overcome some common relationship issues so that you and your partner can get back on the track heading to the land of sexual satisfaction. Do you know the one single thing that turns all men on? Do you know the best way to put the spark back into a sexless relationship? Know what to do when he can't get it up? Do you know the easiest way to destroy your sex life and how you can avoid it? If not, you will soon.

And, for those of you who like things a bit more wild—or think you would like to spice things up, we're also going to cover all of those taboo topics that make most women blush such as sex toys, masturbation, and threesomes. We'll also dive into tantric sex and bondage. So, hang on. It's going to be one wild ride. And, after we're done, you'll be ready to enjoy a really wild ride of your own!

1. *He Likes It When You Get Loud*

Being vocal during sex is a real challenge for some women. But just think about this for a minute. If you're feeling too shy or embarrassed to moan and groan, how much are you holding back on your orgasms? The trick to really amazing sex is to simply let go and one of the easiest ways to do this is to vocalize your passion during sex.

If you're too shy to completely let go in front of him, practice vocalizing your pleasure while he's not there. It's easier than you think.

Also, practice breathing. Too many women hold their breath during sex and that keeps the energy from flowing through their bodies. Breathing and moaning allow that energy to flow. You'll be amazed at how much easier it is to reach orgasm with this simple technique. So, the next time you have sex, lose your inhibitions and scream like a porn star! (You may just want to warn your partner first so he doesn't call the doctor.)

2. *Having More Sex Boosts Your Libido*

Satisfying sex (especially sex that ends in orgasm) just makes you feel good. Why? Well, sex has been shown to raise the level of endorphins—neurotransmitters that reduce pain and increase pleasure—produced in the brain while also reducing stress. So, having more sex makes you feel better and feeling better makes you want sex more often. Why wouldn't you want to do something that makes you feel good?

In fact, a minister in Grapevine, Texas, recently challenged his entire congregation to have sex for seven days straight, and then report the results back to him the following week. Guess what, all who participated felt better and wanted sex more often! So, why not take the seven-day challenge?

Unfortunately, the reverse of this phenomenon is true as well: If you're not having sex, chances are that you've found your libido dragging a bit. So if you haven't had sex in a while, just do it.

HE **SAYS** . . .

If you're in the not-having-sex-very-much rut, break that vicious cycle! Try having sex every day for a week and notice the changes in your physical and emotional state, as well as the intimacy of your relationship. Come on ladies, you'll be helping your man out; this can provide great relief for his right hand, lessening the risk of repetitive stress injury.

3. *Porn Can Turn You On Too*

Men are typically visual creatures and love to sit back and watch all of the nitty-gritty details. However, while men are likely to be turned on by the sight of strange couples and threesomes cavorting on staged sets, many women feel threatened by the carved bodies, pretty faces, and the practiced capabilities of the porno queens. And, while some women love what is typically called *guy porn*, some women prefer erotica.

What is the difference between guy porn and erotica? Well, *erotica* refers to softer images of, and especially writings about, sex. The characters may be model-attractive, but are just as likely to look like ordinary people. Erotica may be explicit in its depiction or description of sex, but is just as likely to involve the more mundane sex almost all of us are lucky to enjoy once or twice a week.

Erotica, in its written form, ranges from raunchy *Penthouse Forum* anecdotes of frat-house sex to literary erotica complete with beautifully crafted sentences, fascinating characters, and zingy plots.

A good starting place for bringing porn into your love life is to find a film that has a bit of a story and some character development. Even if it's cheesy—and your man can share a laugh or two with you about that—you might just find it easier to get into the sex scenes if they have some context. That's essentially how romance novels are written, with sexual scenes strung together with a compelling narrative. The most successful and widely read stories and novels are those involving strong female protagonists engaged in romantic relationships. The sex takes place in the context of those relationships.

*Sex*MYTH: **Women Don't Like Porn (at Least Not Good Girls)** Totally not true! Many women enjoy porn on a regular basis—just typically not the same way that men do. Most women tend to like girl porn that slowly warms up to the more steamy sex scenes and has some sort of storyline. Men tend to enjoy getting straight to the action. Try to find something that you both enjoy or take turns selecting the movie. The important thing to realize is that you do not have to be like the porn stars in looks or actions. Check your brain (and your insecurities) at the door and have fun!

So, if you don't like watching two (or more) people screw on screen, find some form of erotica that really does it for you. Maybe it's a steamy romance novel that only hints at intercourse, or a more detailed romance novel that goes into the details of how, when, and where the hero takes his heroine. Maybe it's a BDSM novel. (By the way, BDSM stands for Bondage & Discipline / Domination & Submission / Sadism & Masochism. More on that later.) If it works for you, who cares what it is!

You can even find erotic videos if you look hard enough. (Most are available on Amazon for discreet shipping. So what are you waiting for?) Here are twenty personal favorites to get you started:

1. *9½ Weeks*
2. *Wild Orchid*
3. *Sliver*
4. *9 Songs (Unrated Full Uncut Version)*
5. *Lie with Me*
6. *Gia (Unrated Edition)*
7. *Poison Ivy: The New Seduction*
8. *Zandalee*
9. *Showgirls*
10. *Original Sin (Unrated Version)*
11. *Embrace of the Vampire*
12. *Basic Instinct—Director's Cut (Ultimate Edition)*
13. *Eyes Wide Shut (Unrated Edition)*
14. *Wild Things*
15. *Swimming Pool (Unrated Version)*
16. *Femme Fatale*
17. *Malena*
18. *Irreversible*
19. *Crash*
20. *Bound*

Chances are the sexy scenes in these films will help you find just the right level of lust and romance to put yourself in a seductive state of mind. That way your man won't have to work so hard and you'll be able to start the action with less down time.

So, take a bath, relax, unwind with your girl porn, and get yourself so warmed up that when your man walks in the door, you simply *have* to do it right then and there. And remember, you don't have to enjoy the same things that your man enjoys, but give girl porn and erotica a try. It really does work!

HE **SAYS . . .**

You should know that men would love to sit down and watch porn with their ladies! There are more couple-friendly alternatives to the mechanical porn flicks that may appeal better to you and still be interesting to him. Honestly, guys will pretty much watch any type of porn that you want if they get to watch it with you.

4. *Let Go of Your Past to Heat Up Your Present*

Though we'd all prefer this not be the case, most couples have to deal with the emotional baggage left over from their partners' previous relationships. How do you deal with the vast array of emotions that surface because of the last guy you lived with or the last girl he loved? What happens when these feelings are negative and self-destructive?

Whether you're in your first or your fiftieth serious relationship, feelings of jealousy ("Why does he still have lunch with her? He should know how that makes me feel!") and insecurity ("His previous girlfriends were all much thinner than I am. I wonder if he thinks I'm fat? He must only be with me until he can find a girl he's really attracted to.") can cause a lot of stress. Part of your worry is wrapped up in your desire to have control over how your partner acts, especially if you feel that he might not act in accordance with your own standards and needs.

HE **SAYS** . . .

A quick tip: If you are feeling jealous, ask yourself if your partner truly gave you reason to doubt his commitment to you. Is he playing games to try and make you jealous, or could it be that something from the past is rearing its head and making you afraid your guy could leave or cheat?

Dealing with It

So what do you need to know? Well, you need to realize that you cannot control your partner. He is an independent being with free will, and worrying about the hidden meanings behind his words or what he is doing when you're not around will only drive you crazy and drive him away. Today, the fact that people sometimes feel as though they own their partners is the real reason behind the fear, anger, jealousy, and insecurity that many people may experience. The best thing to do is to just allow other people to be themselves and love them for who they are and not who you want them to be. After all, unconditional acceptance from your partner—both in and out of the bedroom—is a great aphrodisiac for both of you.

Let It Go

Here's a little tip: By accepting that your partner has had lovers before you and by letting go of any jealousy and insecurity that you have tied to that or tied to your own experiences in past relationships, you can move on and reap the benefits of your present relationship. Perhaps your partner learned a great position or two from a former sexual escapade or he grasped how to overcome some emotional or sexual issues within that relationship so you don't have to now be burdened with them. All of this knowledge and experience will benefit *you* in the bedroom as you're treated to a more skilled partner who understands his own needs and who can better address yours.

5. Position Yourself for Pleasure: Try Girl on Top (Reverse)

The standard Girl on Top position is where your man lies on his back while you straddle him. This position gives you control over the depth of penetration, the angle of penetration (you can angle his penis perfectly to hit your G-spot while thrusting), and even the speed at which you progress. It also allows you to angle your body so that you can rub your clitoris along his pubic bone for added stimulation.

The reversed Girl on Top position is simply Girl on Top with you facing away from your partner. Have your man lay on his back while you straddle him facing his legs. As with the standard Girl on Top position, you have all the control over the depth and angle of penetration, plus he has full view of your bottom. The minor difference here is that instead of being able to rub your clitoris on his pubic bone, you'll have full access to use your hands or your favorite sex toy.

6. *Men Like Women Who Know What They Want*

A little-known fact is that the single-biggest turn-on for most men is a sexually confident woman. Men love when a woman knows what she wants and is not afraid to let them know what that is. It can be incredibly frustrating for a man to have to guess what his woman likes sexually, what turns her on, how to make her orgasm. Well, you can make your partner the happiest man alive—and increase your chances of getting off—simply by letting him know what you want, like, and need, and by sharing those things with him in a loving and sexy manner. And, it never hurts to initiate—it takes some of the pressure off him and lets him know you're more game for sex than he previously thought. Not sure how to strut your sexual confidence? Follow these simple rules:

- Next time you are feeling horny, tell him.
- Wake him up in the middle of the night for a quickie.
- During intercourse, massage your nipples and clitoris— remember men love to watch!
- Wear something incredibly sexy on your next date.
- Go without a bra—or wear one that lets your nipples poke out.
- Go down on him—without making him ask for it.
- Feel free to surprise him—if he's washing dishes, come up behind him and make his night just a little bit better.

- Send him an e-mail (to his personal account) or text message to let him know what he can look forward to once he gets home.
- Tell him what you want in bed—harder, faster, slower, a little to the right.

As you verbalize your sexual needs and act on your sexual impulses, you will not only help your partner discover what really gets your juices flowing, you will make him more eager to please you because he'll be more confident that he can turn you on.

*Sex*MYTH: **If You're Really in Love, You Should Just Know How to Please Your Partner** Nothing could be farther from the truth! What makes a really good lover is a woman (or man) who knows how to communicate with her (or his) partner. What will please your partner is to tell him or, better yet, show him what really turns you on.

7. Clothe Yourself in Confidence

The way you dress can dramatically affect your mood—and whether or not you feel in the mood. Always make sure to wear clothes that fit properly, are free from excessive wear and tear, and make you feel good when you're wearing them.

Clothing that is too tight can make you feel self conscious of your sexy curves, rolls, and dimples. Show them off, but make sure you're confident in whatever you're wearing. Never buy clothes expecting to fit into them soon. That never happens; it's usually a waste of money, no matter how good the deal seemed to be. Also, avoid the temptation to come home and throw on your baggy sweat pants and shirt. Opt for a sexier option that's still comfortable like yoga pants and a cami, or a clingy sun dress. Those items are just as comfortable, but still make you look and feel sexy.

Clothing that is old and worn drains your energy. Go through your closet and throw away (or donate) everything that you haven't worn for the last twelve months. Stop holding onto those old clothes that may or may not come back into style, or that you may or may not ever fit into again. Give them away to someone who can use them right now. Also get rid of, or mend, anything that's ripped or torn.

Remember, if you feel confident and sexy in everything you wear, it will show and your man won't be able to keep his hands to himself.

HE **SAYS . . .**

Let's be honest here. There is nothing that turns a guy on more than a confident, sexy woman. And if you're not feeling it, chances are, your guy's not feeling you. So, get rid of any clothing that doesn't make you feel great and make room in your closet for clothes you *do* love. The ripped and worn ones should go straight in the trash—seriously, just do it—and all the wearable items in there should be collected in a box or plastic bag to be donated to a local charity. Remember, the only baggy sweatshirt your guy wants to see you in, is one of his.

8. *Don't Sabotage Your Sex Life*

Sex is supposed to be fun and, while it's important to take responsibility for making sure that your sex life stays interesting, trying too hard can actually backfire.

What happens when you try too hard to bring back the spark that's faded? Well, you forget to play and have fun. You start holding yourself and your partner to ridiculous standards and expecting him to behave in a certain way. When he doesn't play along, you'll usually end up in a fight.

HE **SAYS . . .**

Have you seen those bad movie scenes where a couple tries and tries and tries to get pregnant? They try so hard that sex becomes a mechanical chore, no longer fun or intimate or at all enjoyable. It's funny to watch on TV, but not as much fun in real life. Keep your sex life fun . . . and don't let this happen to you!

When things get tense in the bedroom—or you feel like you're trying too hard—you know it's time to relax. Play a game, give your partner a massage, try some role-play, just do anything to get out of the place that you're currently in and rekindle the lust that you know you both feel.

9. *Tantric Sex Will Blow Your Mind*

When you think of tantric sex your thoughts may jump to intense sex sessions that are solely for the pursuit of intense pleasure. While much of tantra does involve these kinds of sexual practices—after all, that's what it became known for in the Western world—tantra involves so much more than pure physical pleasure. For example, did you know that tantra is often used as a means of emotional, physical, and spiritual healing, as well as a method for achieving the ultimate intimacy that can exist between two people?

Intrigued? Then read on to discover how tantra can lead you and your partner on the path to ultimate sexual healing and spiritual unity!

Walk the Tantric Path to Healing and Unity

It's no secret that many people have emotional and mental baggage, thanks to previous relationships or life experiences. Not surprisingly, these problems often manifest themselves during particularly intimate moments, including time spent in the bedroom. Whether the problems come from inner issues (perhaps from low self-confidence or body hate) or outer influences (maybe you or your partner experienced abuse or grew up in a loveless household), these mental and emotional scars don't have to become obstacles in your quests for ultimate intimacy.

In fact, tantra is widely known for its healing powers. If you and your partner engage in tantric lovemaking practices, you'll soon find that you both will grow to become more confident, loving, and intimate partners.

Keep It Distinguished

When using tantra in an effort to connect with your partner on an intimate level, it's important to distinguish these nights from normal sack sessions; a healing tantric session shouldn't have the same feel as a normal night of lovemaking. Rather, a healing tantric session will focus more on unleashing and clearing away any mental and emotional obstacles that you or your partner may have in regard to sex and intimacy.

In a healing session, you must first distinguish your role as either Healer or Receiver; for example, if your partner is the one experiencing emotional or mental obstacles to tantric bliss, then you should be the Healer, and he the Receiver. Additionally, it's important to verbally confirm your role with your partner, as this will serve to relax you both in regard to any expectations.

Find a Space

Once each of your roles has been established, set up a comfortable and nonthreatening space in a spot that is familiar to your partner; healing sessions are often successful in the bedroom, as this is usually a space that signifies positive emotions brought about by intimate and relaxing activities. Let your partner know that anything that happens in the space will stay there; this will make him feel more comfortable sharing intimate and vulnerable moments with you. Have him lie down and begin the healing session with a relaxing massage.

This should differ greatly from a massage that's given in the pursuit of pleasure. The healing massage should, rather, focus on massaging nonsexual areas before centering on the different energy channels located in the pelvic region and the heart. Once your partner has expressed his permission for you to move on to the pelvic region, use slow and deliberate massaging movements. Remember, the goal of this activity is not arousal, so don't rush your partner into orgasm; rather, let him experience the different emotions and sensations that come to the surface. For example, if he begins to become aroused or even yells with anxiety, let him feel these emotions.

Of course, if your partner wishes for you to stop, then the healing session should immediately end until he is ready to begin again. Sometimes, past experiences can be so painful that it can definitely take more than one tantric healing session to release these roadblocks to pleasure and intimacy.

Practice Makes Perfect!

If you desire to play the role of Healer but feel uncomfortable with what it entails, try enrolling in a tantric healing course before engaging in these practices with your lover.

An expert can teach you what to do and how to react in certain scenarios, especially those in which powerful emotions come to the surface. An expert can also help you to become more in touch with your Receiver's energy, which will help you immensely during your healing sessions.

After each tantric healing session, be sure that you hold and nurture your partner, as this will reassure him of your love and devotion to his physical, mental, and emotional well-being. Drink water, take a bath together, or just lie there holding each other, listening to each other's breath.

Soon, your healing sessions will give way to more soulful and sensual lovemaking sessions, as you and partner will have overcome any obstacles to spiritual, physical, and emotional bliss and intimacy.

10. He'll Love Your Lingerie—Especially If You Show It Off Before You Buy It

Buying lingerie can be frustrating, especially if you're by yourself trying to guess what he'll like and won't like, wondering if it looks good on you, etc. Next time, take him with you to the store and let him pick out the lingerie. It can be an eye-opening experience! You may be surprised at what he chooses, but go in with an open mind and buy the outfit that he likes.

Make sure to visit the more upscale stores. They'll actually let you go into the dressing room together so that you can model your potential new purchases. That way you'll know that you've bought something that he loves. If he likes it enough, you may not even make it out of the dressing room.

For some added spice, wear your new purchase under your clothes when you leave the store. He'll have the image of you in your new lingerie for the rest of the day!

11. *He Likes How You Smell . . . Down There*

This may come as a complete shock to you, but men love the natural odor of your vagina. When aroused, men and women release chemicals known as pheromones that let the opposite sex know they're in the mood. And, one of the places that these pheromones are emitted the strongest is in the vaginal area. Once released, they circulate near that area and become trapped in the pubic hair. So, since it's no wonder that he enjoys your natural scent, you don't have to be nervous about him going down on you—and when you're not nervous, it will be much easier for you to lay back and enjoy the ride—and the subsequent orgasm.

Something Smells Fishy

Now, while men do love the natural smell of a woman, a day or two of not showering can make him change his mind about whether or not he's going to pleasure you down below with his tongue. So, if you're on a camping trip or somewhere else you know you'll be without the bathing conveniences of home, but still want to have a free sexual experience, bring along some baby wipes so you can freshen up! On a more serious note, if you notice that your vaginal area has been smelling off, you may want to think about calling your doctor as you might have a yeast infection or other vaginal condition that needs addressing.

12. *Have an Affair (with Him)*

Listen. It's been said again and again that variety is the spice of life. Don't let boredom kill your relationship or your sex life. If you've been with your partner for more that a few months, you may have gotten into a sexual rut. You've found what's comfortable and what seems to work for one another sexually and it can be scary to change anything. But the main reason that many couples stop having sex is that it just gets boring.

*Sex*MYTH: **If He Had an Affair That Means You're Not Good in Bed** *Affairs and cheating are rarely about the sex.* Read that last sentence until you really get it. Most people have affairs when they are feeling emotionally disconnected from their partners— unappreciated, unsupported, misunderstood, etc. Cheating and affairs are only symptoms of deeper issues in relationships. If you work together to resolve these deeper issues in your relationship, there will be no affair. Period.

When your sex life becomes routine or monotonous that is when you or your partner may begin to wonder "What was I thinking?"

You may start to reminisce about what it was like in the beginning of the relationship—exciting, new, and spontaneous. Thoughts of having an affair start to come up. Maybe that's the answer to a boring sex life—someone new!

Stop right there!

HE **SAYS . . .**

We don't want to get stuck in a rut either ladies! We loved those days where we didn't know what you'd be wearing until we knocked on your door or when we weren't sure you wanted to be kissed until you made the first move. We never want to stop dating! Remember what you and your partner used to do when you first got together: paying special attention to one another, going on frequent dates, kissing, etc. Keep doing those things every day. It'll make your relationship stronger and your sex life more intense.

How about having an affair with your partner? Add some newness and adventure to your current relationship. Spice things up. Try some role-play. Have an affair with your partner—as long as he's willing. The following are some ideas to get you started.

Send a Naughty E-mail

Send an e-mail to your lover from a private e-mail account. The initial e-mail should be flirty and suggestive, but don't move too fast. Remember, you are strangers trying to get to know one another better. You should both create a new e-mail account for this purpose. You can even create whole new identities. Be someone that you wish you were but are afraid to be.

Meet in Secret

Once you've developed an interest in one another over e-mail (or IM/Chat), arrange a secret meeting for lunch or drinks. Keep a low profile and don't get caught. Don't tell anyone what you're doing or, even better, tell your best friend or coworker that you've met this incredible guy—and watch the rumors fly! Even though you're doing this with your partner, it should be adventurous and exciting. It should feel wrong (without being wrong).

Create Rules

The one rule is that you can never have your affair at home. Part of the fun is finding new and exciting places to hook up. You can keep this affair going as long as you like and, when you're ready to try something new, you can even invent a breakup and then reinvent yourselves again, or pretend to get married and enjoy the honeymoon phase of your relationship again.

The important thing is to never stop dating and never stop looking for fun ways to invigorate your relationship and your sex life. As soon as it gets too comfortable, it's time to play!

13. Position Yourself for Pleasure: Try the Cross

This is a great position for you because it gives you more control of the angle of your legs and hips—unlike some other man-on-top positions where you don't have as much mobility. In addition, with this position your entire body, from your breasts to your clitoris, is exposed for extra stimulation. It's a great position for your man to make use of a clitoral vibrator or bullet; the extra stimulation will send you over the edge. To get into the Cross position, lie on your back with your legs slightly spread. Your partner should lie diagonally across from you. You should then place your legs over the top of your partner's hips for penetration. You can improve the angle of penetration even more by placing a few pillows under your bottom or rotating your hips to the left or right. Once you find the perfect angle, this is guaranteed to be one of your favorite positions

14. *Learn to Touch Yourself—and Then Teach Your Man Your Moves*

This is one of those topics that seems so simple and is yet so taboo even in this modern age. Why are so many women afraid to masturbate? Why are they too shy to talk about it or to touch themselves in front of or with their partners?

SexMYTH: Most Women Orgasm Through Intercourse

Actually, most women orgasm through a combination of clitoral and vaginal stimulation, instead of vaginal stimulation alone, because there are many more nerves within the clitoris than within the vagina.

Think about it. How on earth can you have a satisfying and enjoyable sex life if you don't even know what you like? How can you tell your partner how to please you, if you don't know what gets you off? Remember, he's not psychic.

If you don't masturbate already, put this book down and go touch yourself. It doesn't matter if you know what you're doing or not, just take off your clothes and look at yourself in the mirror. Then try touching various parts of your body to see what feels good and what doesn't.

Most women orgasm from stimulation of the clitoris, but others can only orgasm from vaginal penetration (also known as G-spot stimulation). However, there is no wrong or right way to masturbate because everyone responds differently. Give it a try and see what works for you. It's easier than you think.

How to Masturbate

Before you masturbate, make sure to relax and get comfortable. A good way to do this is to take a shower or bath. Then, when you get out, rub lotion all over your body; just take your time and move slowly. Pay attention to the areas that are more responsive and easily aroused. Try touching your vagina, nipples, inner and outer labia, clitoris, perineum, or even your stomach and inner thighs.

As you become more aroused, you may want to lie down or sit down so that you're more relaxed. Keep massaging the area that brings you the most pleasure and don't forget to breathe! Breathing deeply is very important during orgasm. It allows your sexual energy to flow. If you hold your breath, you block this energy.

When you feel an orgasm coming, continue stimulating yourself until the orgasm is finished. If you don't have an orgasm on your first try, keep practicing. Remember, practice makes perfect!

Once you are comfortable masturbating and reaching orgasm, you can begin to experiment with sex toys such as vibrators and dildos to increase your pleasure and increase the ease and strength of your orgasms.

Mutual Masturbation

Here's a twist on masturbation that you should try. Mutual masturbation with your partner can be very erotic, and showing him that side of you can create intimacy and bring you closer. Just remember, he is showing you that side of him too!

If you are a little shy, start on the sofa, under a blanket with your favorite adult movie playing on the TV. You don't even have to talk about it; just the idea of you touching yourself under the blanket will drive him wild! Once you're feeling a little more comfortable, you can pull the blanket away and let him watch. There are few things that turn a man on more than watching his woman please herself!

Oh, one more point on this topic. Women can be so critical of their bodies and it's completely unjustified. Love yourself and be grateful for who you are and what you have. Self-loathing has been linked to a whole myriad of diseases and conditions and it makes perfect sense. It doesn't matter if you are a size 2 or a size 20—when you look at yourself in the mirror, look yourself in the eyes and say out loud, "I love you. You are a beautiful person." Do it every day until you really mean it—starting right now.

What you focus on grows! This is true whether you focus on the good or the bad. So love yourself first!

15. Try Some Kinky, Freaky Sex

A friend of mine told me about something embarrassing and awkward that happened to her when she was having sex with her partner. They were having really great, spur-of-the-moment sex when he grabbed her wrists and held them over her head. My friend was surprised—and emotionally uncomfortable—and told her partner as much.

HE **SAYS** . . .

Trust me when I tell you that many men love kinky, freaky sex even if they won't admit it. This, for example, is why we're seeing anal sex becoming so popular; in most cases it's the guy's fantasy. Men like to push the forbidden envelope, and do what they're not really supposed to do. Although, frankly, down deep, so do women, you're just not usually as open and vocal about it.

They decided to keep going and talked about it after they both finished. My friend told her partner that his actions made her feel embarrassed and confused. She said it made her feel out of control and like he was just using her for sex. She needed to feel nurtured and loved and instead she felt like an object. Her partner told her that he did what he felt was right in the moment. To him it was an incredibly instinctive gesture that he did to make sex a little better, a little wilder. He didn't really think that she would react the way she did because the motion felt so right at the time. But there you have it—that one simple grab of the wrist made her uncomfortable and pushed her boundaries.

Most people are so naturally hypocritical about sexual preferences. Whatever they're comfortable with is *normal* and whatever they're not yet comfortable with is *weird* or *kinky*. The trick is to understand that everyone sees sexuality in their own unique and special ways. And once you open up to your partner about your wants, desires, and fantasies, you open up a very special connection in your relationship. Wouldn't it be awesome to find out that you and your partner share some of the same fantasies and desires? That would mean they wouldn't have to be secret—or just fantasies—anymore.

But to do that, you have to be open and willing to trying new experiences with your partner—even if they make you uncomfortable at first. Be willing to release your inhibitions and let go of your sexual baggage. This will open the doorway to incredible sexual experiences that you never dreamt were possible.

16. *The Way to a Man's Heart (and Other Parts of His Anatomy) Really Is Through His Stomach*

Here's the thing. Every guy was once a boy and the first woman who ever loved—or fed—him was his mother. When a woman cooks for a man, it provides him with a certain warmth and comfort. By cooking for him, you are taking the time to care, nurture, and nourish him. These qualities are vital for men looking for a long-term relationship.

HE **SAYS . . .**

Remember how special time together seemed when you first met, when you were first dating? Do those little things that felt special back then, and it may just shock you what a difference it makes to your relationship.

Rather than going out for dinner, cook his favorite meal and set the mood with soft lighting and candles. To add some extra spice, make sure he is there while you are cooking in nothing but an apron.

Don't like to cook? Order in and feed him with your fingers. Remember, men love to be nurtured and feeding him can be an incredibly sexy way to nurture, especially if you're naked.

17. Scheduled Sex Can Be Great Sex

We know you're tired, exhausted even. Of course you've had a really long day.

But whether your relationship is two weeks or twenty years old, it's critical to nurture it and make time for one another—and for sex. Schedule some time to just be together: Whether it's first thing in the morning, after a nice lunch, or some quiet couple time before you drift off to sleep, couple time is very important. Also, if you know your day is going to have a happy ending, you'll be hot to trot as soon as you walk in the door! If that doesn't make your sex life better, I don't know what will. So, get out your calendar and make a date!

*Sex*MYTH: **You Shouldn't Plan Sex** It depends! While falling into the same routine night after night can be dull—and this goes for more than just sex—planning a night of fun with your partner doesn't mean it won't be a blast. In fact, it can be even more exciting than spontaneous sex as you can plan to wear your sexiest lingerie, pick up some fun aphrodisiacs . . . well, you get the picture. And, especially with those of us who have busy schedules, making sure we make the time to have sex is important!

18. De-Stress for Amazing Sex

Stress is the biggest enemy of your health—especially your sexual health. Job stress, financial stress, life stress (feeling overwhelmed), and especially relationship stress can all have negative effects on your health and reduce your libido. After all, it's hard to get in the mood if you can't stop your mind from thinking about that report you need to finish at work or whether you need to schedule a babysitter for Saturday night. There's no reason to live with stress. So, here are five easy ways to reduce your stress levels—and lift your libido—in just fifteen minutes or less:

1. **Meditate/Breathe:** Breathe deeply. It seems in our busy hectic society we have forgotten how to breathe. Spend 5–10 minutes just breathing. Sit in a comfortable position, close your eyes, and breathe with your diaphragm.

   - Inhale as deeply as you can (your stomach should expand if you're doing this correctly) for a slow count of 8–16. Completely fill your lungs starting from the top and expanding deep into your chest.
   - Hold your breath for 4–8 counts.
   - Exhale slowly starting from the bottom of your lungs and working to the top for 8–16 counts.
   - Hold your empty lungs for 4–8 counts.
   - Repeat at least ten times.

2. **Take a Walk:** Whether your stress is work-related or you're fighting with your partner, politely excuse yourself and talk a brisk walk around the block (or the parking lot).

3. **Enjoy a Cup of Tea:** Make yourself a soothing cup of your favorite tea. Caffeine-free, herbal tea is best for relaxation, but the most important thing is that you enjoy the tea and the experience. Breathe in the aroma and slowly sip the tea, be in the moment and focus on relaxing.

4. **Stretch:** Get up and stretch! Start from your head and work all the way down your body.

- Roll your neck slowly from side to side.
- Roll your shoulders to the front and to the back.
- Reach up as high as you can and lift up onto your toes.
- Come down and bend over slowly letting your hands hang toward the ground. Don't worry about reaching the floor, just relax and breathe deeply (in and out) several times.
- Roll up slowly and reach for the sky. Repeat this reaching and bending sequence several times until you feel relaxed.

5. **Get a Massage:** While an hour massage is preferred, getting a fifteen minute chair massage is far better than nothing!

19. *Turn Your Fantasies into Reality*

Everyone has fantasies—and some have more than others. Many people choose not to act out their fantasies; afraid they'll embarrass themselves or offend their partners. But how can you achieve a truly deep bond with your partner if you're holding in your deepest desires?

HE **SAYS . . .**

My best advice for a long-term, successful relationship is to live it one day at a time. If you can say before you go to bed each night "I want to see you again tomorrow," then you're well on your way to a life-long relationship, one day at a time.

When it comes to acting out fantasies, as long as your fantasy is safe (as in, it won't cause anyone harm) and is between consenting adults, there's no reason you shouldn't be able to enjoy yourselves and have fun! How can you tell if your partner is sexually compatible with you and your fantasy without putting yourself out there and risking embarrassment? The trick is *not* to have a sit-down talk with your partner. Often, this can be overwhelming, especially if your fantasy is something he's never had any experience with before.

Try introducing your partner to your fantasy slowly, by dressing in some lingerie or a costume that suits your fantasy, or even simply playing with dominant and submissive roles. If your partner shows that he is interested in the fantasy that you're showing him, or turned on by what you're doing, try introducing a little more each time until you're really ready to tell them about what you want to act out and what your total fantasy is.

The bottom line is, as long as your fantasy is between consenting adults, you can have fun indulging in your sexual desires and grow closer to your partner by doing it.

20. *Buying a Sex Toy Is Not as Scary as You Think*

Buying your first sex toy can be an intimidating experience. Where do you start? How do you know what you'll like? Are they expensive?

To make it easy, here are five simple questions that you should answer to help you choose the perfect sex toy for you. Trust us, it's easier than you think it is!

Question #1 How Are You Going to Use Your Sex Toy?

The first step is to decide how you're going to use a prospective sex toy. Ask yourself these questions:

- Do I want to use it by myself?
- Do I want to use it with a partner?
- Do I want to try both?
- Do I need a vibrator with titillating action, or will a non-vibrating, standard dildo be sufficient?
- Do I want something just to massage my clitoris, or would I like to use it for insertion?
- Do I want a toy that does double-duty and both massages my clitoris and inserts and stimulates my G-spot at the same time?

Deciding what the most important aspects of owning a sex toy are for you is a crucial first step in finding the vibrator that suits your needs.

Question #2 What Material Do You Want Your Sex Toy to Be Made Out Of?

There are several different types of sex-toy materials available on the market today; for example, one of the newer materials is called Cyberskin and is soft and squishy, with a very realistic skin-like sensation. This is a great material for a penis-shaped dildo, making it more realistic. You can also buy plastic, silicone, or steel vibrators, or go with softer silicone or even glass dildos or vibrators. Check out a sex toy website that will allow you to browse the different materials that are available so you can find out what type of material intrigues you the most.

Question #3 What Size and Shape Should Your Sex Toy Be?

Size and shape are very important when it comes to finding the perfect sex toy or dildo for you. Vibrators and dildos come in a complete variety of shapes and sizes. Do you want something small and discreet that will fit in your handbag? Or would you prefer a very large, very wide dildo that will bring you the maximum amount of pleasure that you can withstand? Do you want something medium-sized that will get the job done? Think about what you're most comfortable with sexually so you can find the right size for you; it's not a one-size-fits-all sort of deal.

Question #4 What Do You Prefer for Your Vibrator's Power Source?

If you've decided to go with a vibrator and not a standard dildo (it's easy to remember which is which: vibrators vibrate, dildos don't), you can run into the issues of having to stop what you're doing to recharge your vibrator or switch batteries. Both are good ways to power your vibrator, but both have their disadvantages. Running out of batteries (and not having any more on hand) in the heat of the moment can be a huge disappointment, while having a cordless, rechargeable vibrator can be quite expensive. Think about how convenient you want your vibrator to be by determining how often you think you're going to use it.

Question #5 How Much Do You Want to Spend?

Keep in mind that you get what you pay for. If this is your first vibrator or dildo, you might not be prepared to spend a hundred dollars or more on the hottest, most realistic vibrator on the market today. But that doesn't mean there isn't a middle ground. Look for a dildo or vibrator that is in your price range, but realize that the cheaper you go, the less features and power your new vibrator will have.

21. *The Kitchen Can Be Kinky Too*

For most people, the kitchen is the heart of the home and people gather there to eat, drink, and make merry. But that's not all that can happen in there . . . since the kitchen is such a perfect, welcoming, together place, you might as well screw there too! Unfortunately, most lovers never take the opportunity to fully explore all of the hidden erotic treasures awaiting them in their kitchen drawers because they are too busy focusing on food to spend several savory hours indulging their sensual sides.

What do we suggest? Plan a date night with your lover, but, instead of having a night out on the town, make the kitchen your destination. Put as much effort into getting ready as you would for any other date and make arrangements so you won't be bothered with any distractions, be it your kids, your pet, or your cell phones.

Start the date by opening the refrigerator and cabinets and looking for items that could be used in sensual ways. Soon, everything from the baster to the butter will be inspiring you to try out some new, kinky ideas and you'll never think of that once-dull whisk or spatula the same way again. To get you started on your delicious journey, here are five common items that can be secretly used for fun sexual play.

The Wooden Spoon

Have you ever been baking and given your partner a smack on the bottom or the shoulder with a wooden spoon? Come on, admit it. You know you have at least thought of letting one fly. A wooden spoon is an ideal replacement for a paddle, and is much less expensive! It will give your partner's behind a nice little sting, but won't hurt too much—and if it does, feel free to soothe the pain with some newly sexy items from the fridge. (Maybe ice, chocolate, butter, or even frozen peas!) Plus, for those who like the idea of spanking, a wooden spoon makes a really nice, solid whacking sound.

Food Play

Chocolate is an obvious option for food play—melt it in the microwave or in a double broiler on the stove and use your fingers to draw chocolate lines on your partner that you can then slowly and seductively lick off. Then, use a kitchen brush to paint chocolate onto the body parts you want your partner to lick and encourage him to indulge.

22. *Position Yourself for Pleasure: Give Him a Lap Dance*

We're sure you've heard of, and have maybe even given your partner, a lap dance or strip tease, but using the lap dance as a sexual position brings the dance to a new level—and puts you in control. To try it out, straddle your partner while he sits in a chair. You can either face him or face away, but whatever direction you choose, you should keep your knees at his sides and spread wide. You can then move up, down, and around in a rhythmic motion until both you and your partner come.

While this may seem like a dance for your partner, you will receive the pleasure of being able to control the angle and depth of penetration as well as the speed at which intercourse progresses. If he gets too far ahead of you, you can simply walk away until he calms down a bit. Plus, if you choose the right chair, like one of those armless desk chairs, you can adjust the height and use the back for added support. Some of them even lean back a little. Just be careful that you don't end up on the floor unexpectedly!

23. Guys Like Girls Who Give Good Head

Oral sex is one of the most intimate gifts you can give your partner, so why not become really good at giving the gift? Here are some tips that will help you master this critical skill.

Remember, You're in Charge

When you go down on your guy, you are the one giving him pleasure; therefore, you are the one making the choices. You are not obligated in any way to do any particular action or technique that makes you uncomfortable. Your man may tend to grab onto your head during oral sex, or start thrusting in your mouth. If you enjoy this, then have fun, but don't feel that you have to do it simply because it brings him pleasure. If you don't like something he's doing, let him know and move on to something you both enjoy.

HE **SAYS . . .**

For most sexual activities, it helps to have mutual understanding of what you both like. (And trust me, guys want to know what the women they're with are into!) And if you're really, really lucky, you may both like the same thing!

Part of what really turns a man on about oral sex (and manual stimulation) is that he is giving up control. So, as you perform any oral or manual technique, make sure that he knows you're in charge and completely confident in your ability to bring him to orgasm on your terms and your timing, and that he can trust you to give him a better orgasm than he's ever had before.

Men Are Visual Creatures

Men love to look. They process a lot of their information directly through their eyes. So, if you want to give your partner an out-of-this-world experience, provide visuals for him. Look him in the eye and use your face to convey your enjoyment of what you are doing and the way he's responding. Position yourself so he can get a good look at you, particularly the areas he's attracted to, such as your breasts or bottom.

Recreate the Vagina

When you are giving manual or oral stimulation, you are basically recreating for your partner the sensation of being inside a vagina—without actually using one. So, what do you need to simulate that experience?

- **Friction and Pressure:** Ideally, vaginas fit snugly around the penis and hug tightly. This translates into the sensations of friction (rubbing) and pressure. For this reason, use a firm grip with your hands or lips and tongue. Make sure to ask him how hard or soft he likes it.
- **Moisture:** An aroused vagina is wet. So, using lubrication on your hands or having saliva in the mouth can help give him that feeling of wetness that will really float his boat.
- **Changing Temperatures:** As the penis moves in and out of the vagina, it experiences alternating sensations of heat and cooling. Again the movement in and out of your mouth can recreate this sensation. You can also use warming lubricants on your hands as well.

Communication Is Key

During any type of sex, communication is critical! It's the only way you can find out what works and what doesn't for both of you.

When he is in the process of getting off, your man will tend to focus on the overall experience (which communication will help you enhance), rather than on the specific techniques that you use. Chances are, when all is said and done, he won't remember exactly what happened, how it happened, or when. The only thing that will stick out in his mind is that it was really good.

*Sex*MYTH: **Men Reach Their Peaks at 18, Women at 28** It's true that these are the gender-specific ages that the hormones peak, but that doesn't mean that a man is any less able to have a great orgasm or be a good lover later in life and it doesn't mean your orgasms will be worse at 29 and beyond. As we age, we become better lovers because we know our own bodies better and have learned more sexual techniques, so don't link peak hormones with peak performance or else you might be sorely disappointed.

Here are some important methods of communication that you can use when giving him something to remember.

Eye Contact

One of the secrets to a great blow job is making eye contact with your lover. After all, when you look at him, you're better able to gauge his responses. This will help you learn what works and what doesn't. Also, by looking at him, you can communicate the pleasure you feel when pleasuring him. This is very important. Knowing that you like going down will help him keep it up.

Facial Expression

Eye contact is important, but you can also use your facial expressions to show how much you are enjoying yourself. Imagine that you are a film actress and that you are a giving a close-up just for him. Before you go down on him, keep in mind that men love to see a woman's lips parted slightly because it shows that you're turned on and want to be kissed . . . or more. And, when you're ready to go further—or even if you're taking a break from going down—a big smile of pure enjoyment can go a long way because it reveals that you too are having fun, which will make it easier for your man to relax into the moment. The important thing is to not simply stare off into space. Let him see that you're enjoying what you're doing!

Body Language

Your body can express a lot just in the way you are sitting or moving. If you lean toward him, you'll convey your desire to be closer to him. If you move back, you can signal your desire to slow down. Your hands speak to him as you touch his body. But don't think you are limited to hands. You have arms, feet, legs, hair, and a torso to work with. Here are some great moves to help you use what you have:

- Throw your head back, arch your back, and stick out your chest while making love.
- Rub your breasts or bottom against him as you pass him in the kitchen.
- Next time you're sitting in a chair across from him, spread your legs—wide open!
- Bend over and show him your sexy bottom the next time you need to pick something up.

- Let him see your cleavage, or better yet, let your nipple accidentally peek out of your shirt.
- Use your foot to massage his crotch while having dinner at your favorite restaurant.

As you can see, the only limit to the ways you can use your body is your own imagination.

Vocalizing

Finally, there is vocalizing. Talking, moaning, and even heavy breathing can convey an infinite number of feelings and emotions. Here are a few ideas for how you can make oral sex more enjoyable with sound:

- Ask him questions. Does he like what you're doing? Does he want more? Ask him to tease you or stimulate you back.
- Tell him what to do. Remember, he's giving control over to you.
- Tease him by telling him what you are planning to do. Don't be afraid to talk; a lot of men love that.
- Praise him, especially his penis. Express your amazement at its size, power, and hardness.
- Remember that verbalization is a two-way street. Allow him the space to express his pleasure at what you are doing.

Lubrication, Lubrication, Lubrication!

Last, but not least, is lubrication. While friction and pressure are important, too much friction can be painful for him. The most natural lubricant for oral sex is saliva, which you produce when your saliva glands are stimulated (as they are when you are hungry and see some delicious food or when you're horny and see a delicious man). However, for other sexual activities, we recommend investing in a good-quality commercial lubricant.

24. *Leave the Lights on for Lustful Lovemaking*

Here's a little secret: He wants to see your body. Sure, *you* might feel insecure about the way this or that looks, but trust us, he is not going to notice. All he's going to notice is that he has a gorgeous, naked woman in bed with him. So, instead of waiting until the lights are off and the room is pitch black to undress, take the time to get undressed—or better yet, have him undress you—while the lights are still on. Not only will it give him a chance to be in awe of your form, it will allow you to admire his as well, which we bet will turn you on. After all, you two likely ended up in bed together because you found each other attractive, so don't get shy now. Being more free and comfortable with your body will allow you to relax and enjoy great sex as you can focus on feeling great instead of being hung up on your insecurities.

Sexy Shadows

Now, while making love in the light is terribly sexy, it depends on the type of light. Natural sunlight is ideal, but if it's nighttime, having a shaded lamp near the bed is perfect because it will create delicate, sensual shadows across your bodies and a more romantic atmosphere. What you want to avoid are any lights that are super bright or harsh—like many ceiling lamps and fluorescents—as you don't want to feel like you're being interrogated when you're having sex.

Romantic Candlelight

If you really want to rev up the Hollywood-romance feel of your lovemaking, we suggest trying candlelight. A few well-placed candles on a nightstand or dresser near the bed certainly add to the mood and will also send flickering shadows dancing across your bodies. Very sexy indeed. When considering whether to purchase scented or unscented candles, consider if there are any scents he is attracted to—for instance, does he always nuzzle your neck if you're wearing a lavender perfume?—and lean toward those scents, especially if they are compelling to you as well. If you're not sure, choose unscented candles just in case.

25. Have Fun with Fetishes

Everyone has a fetish. Yes, even you! You just may not realize that it's a fetish. Here's the deal. You have to come to terms with the fact that everyone is a pervert. That's right—just like how everyone has to use the bathroom, every adult you know is secretly harboring her own brand of kink. Some never utter what truly excites them out loud. Some never share it with their partners. The poor dears are afraid of freaking people out.

HE **SAYS** . . .

Our real kinks are what we secretly think about when masturbating alone in the dark—and yours are too. You don't have to admit it to anyone if you don't want to, but it's important for you to come to terms and be at peace with it.

It would be nice if there was a national coming-out day for fetishes and fantasies, a day where every person would put it right out there on the table and acknowledge her turn-ons. As in: "Hello, my name is Lucy, and I have a thing for werewolves / feet / bondage / etc."

Trust us when we tell you that even the most conservative person has something that titillates her. So fly your freak flag and start to fill your partner in on what gets you off!

Mary, Mary, Quite Contrary, How Does Your Fetish Grow?

I'm a big fan of taking baby steps. If you're afraid to tell your partner about your fetish, plant a little seed and then back off. Don't tell him, "I want to host an orgy." Instead, say something like, "Wouldn't it be hot if there was someone over there in the corner watching us have sex?" or "I think watching two girls kiss is completely sexy; if you had to pick a female celebrity to make out with, who would you choose?"

Until your partner is more comfortable, always include him in your fantasy scenario. If you don't, he will feel threatened and alienated. You want him to feel like he is a part of this intimate thing you are sharing, a partner in crime, if you will. Be patient with him and give him time to digest the idea. Then, slowly up the ante when the timing seems right.

Are You Ready to Come Out?

Sure you are! If you're still feeling shy, you can start by going online and searching for the things that turn you on. The one thing I've heard over and over again from loads of people is: "Thank God for the Internet. I'm not the only one." Join an online community; it feels great to be able to let down your guard and talk openly about what you like, even if it is anonymously.

Next, confess your fetish to a trusted friend, the kind of friend who would pick you up at 3 A.M. if your car broke down, or bring you a care package of cold syrup and cough drops if you were home sick fighting a monster cold.

Finally, open up to the person you are closest to—you know, the one you sleep with. I hear a lot of people claim that they married their best friends, and who is a best friend but someone you can share everything with? As in: no secrets (and no shame). So just open up and see how much fun you'll have when you disclose your deepest, darkest desires to the one who will help you put them into practice.

26. Subtlety Can Be Seductive

The female body is a thing of beauty, and nudity can be very satisfying, but full nudity is rarely involved in true seduction. The fine art of teasing with what is just out of view is a favorite technique employed by the most sought-after sexy ladies.

HE SAYS . . .

Yes! It's not all about full nudity or birdie shots, they're not always the most erotic, most arousing, nor most conducive to setting a man's imagination on fire. What really makes a man burn with desire is the *teasing*, the almost-there peek at something he can't have or see yet!

So how can you tease your man? Well, lingerie and sexy costumes are proven and effective tools used in the art of seduction. Don't feel silly. Take a minute and consider what you dream and fantasize about. Really. What do you think about when no one else is around? Are you a goddess who is worshiped and adored by her lover? Or perhaps a wicked seductress claiming any lover she desires? Stop living your fantasies only in your head. Lingerie and sexy costumes allow you to become anyone you want to be—even if just for a little while.

HE **SAYS . . .**

It may surprise you to know that not all guys like all types of lingerie. Really! It's all about how it looks on their women. After all, it's not the lingerie guys like (or they'd wear it themselves), it's how it looks on you. And if you are comfortable and feel sexy in what you have on, then you'll find your man more than willing to take it off.

So what are the most popular lingerie items that men can't get enough of?

1. **The Chemise:** A chemise is basically a very silky mini-dress. The chemise is not only incredibly sexy, but it's also comfortable, so you're more likely to wear it more often.
2. **The Babydoll:** The babydoll is similar to the chemise but typically has an underwire bra for added cleavage and support. Plus, it has a slit down the middle starting underneath your chest, to reveal your sexy tummy. Oh, and it normally comes with bikini underwear or a thong.
3. **The Teddy:** Think of the teddy as a really sexy one-piece swimsuit with a hole in the crotch. Men love the sexy contours and easy access.

4. **Camisole & Thong:** A simple camisole and thong is always a big hit because you look really sexy wearing it and yet it appears completely innocent and accidental.

5. **Push-up Bra, G-string & Garter Belts:** If you really want to go all-out porn star, this is the proven option. Garter belts and lots of cleavage have been used to seduce men for years and they still work. Oh, and don't forget the screw-me stilettos!

27. Massage Can Be an Aphrodisiac

Sensual massage is one of the best natural aphrodisiacs there is. And the good news? You don't have to be an expert to give a good sensual massage. Here are the basic how-tos for a really great erotic massage:

1. Create a relaxing and sexual environment. This includes dimming the lights, or setting some candles around the room for lighting and aroma. Put clean sheets or blankets on the floor, bed, or massage table. Put on some soft music in the background.

2. Start by massaging your partner's head and face. Run your fingers through his hair and massage his scalp. Massage his temples in circles and gently stroke his forehead by moving from the center out to the temples. Then, gently stroke from the center of his nose, under his cheekbones, and out to his ears. Finally stroke the top of his lips, around his mouth, and to his chin.

3. Have your partner lie face down. Rub your hands together with a good massage oil to warm them and lubricate them. Start by gently kneading his neck and shoulder muscles,

then, using gently gliding strokes, work your way down one arm all the way to the fingertips. You don't have to be extremely firm, but make sure to always have one hand touching your partner; it's startling when the contact is broken. Slowly work back up the arm, across the shoulders, down the other arm, and back up again.

4. Next, make long strokes up and down your partner's back with one hand on each side of the spine. The pressure should be firm but gentle, and you want to avoid working directly over the spine—the last thing you want to do is hurt your partner while you're trying to get him to relax.

5. Gradually work down the back to your partner's bottom. Knead the cheeks, one in each hand. Don't go to his genitals or to the back door—yet—just continue to massage the muscles.

6. Repeat the same long strokes that you practiced on the arms and back down each leg and remember to never lose contact with the skin. Next, hold onto his foot and rotate his ankle in both directions, stretch it front and back, and use your thumbs to massage the underside of his foot. Lastly, gently pull on each of his toes. Work back up his leg slowly and repeat on the other leg.

7. Then, ask you partner to turn over. Massage his arms again from the front. Massage his chest and stomach gently, too. Work all the way down the sides gently to his hips.

8. As you reach his hips, lower stomach, and upper legs, you'll be massaging several erogenous zones. It's not even necessary to directly massage his genitals, but if your partner seems willing you can gently caress or brush against them. This will likely drive him crazy, but (for now) your job is to continue the massage.

9. Massage your partner's legs with long gentle strokes that work down to the feet—just as you did on the backs of the legs. Repeat the foot massage as well. Work your way back to the upper legs.

10. Make sure your partner achieves his happy ending. If your partner is willing, you can return slowly back up the legs, but this time, slowly include the genitals, increasing the pleasure until he reaches the peak of ecstasy.

28. Size Does Matter

Try as we might to tell men that we care more about the motion of the ocean, guys will never listen. For them, it is the size of the boat that counts. Your man may always want more girth or more length, even if you think he's more than adequate. But how large is a normal penis? Well, that's a question that many men ask, especially in conjunction with questions about penis growth, but it's a difficult question to answer. What is normal isn't necessarily classified; all men are different and everyone has different anatomy. No two penises will ever be exactly the same! But generally speaking, the typical penis ranges between 2–3 inches long when it is flaccid and between 5–6 inches when it is hard. Many men, however, fall outside these categories and that doesn't necessarily mean there is anything wrong with them!

Honestly, Does Penis Size Really Matter?

If a penis fits the vagina, it really doesn't matter how big it measures because, well, it fits! Where sexual pleasure is concerned, the greatest pleasure is often derived from intercourse with someone whose genitals physically match your own. But, if the sex feels good to you, then your man's penis is perfect. If you feel the sex could be better, you may need to find ways to work around your man's shortcomings.

Creative Ways to Work a Size Mismatch

If you are mismatched anatomically, don't rely completely on intercourse for you and your partner's sexual pleasure. It will lead to very boring, monotonous sex especially if you two have a size mismatch. Work with your partner to find new and creative ways you can please each other sexually in addition to intercourse. Using a little extra lubrication or a toy during intercourse may stimulate you so much that you won't even be thinking about your partner's penis size. Try incorporating oral sex on both the receiving and giving ends, or use hands and toys to give your partner pleasure. If you stick to just intercourse, you're likely to be frustrated and disappointed.

HE SAYS . . .

The most important thing about penis size is a good fit. Neither too small nor too big is ideal. So many men are afraid of not being big enough, not realizing that guys with huge penises have the opposite problem, which is just as bad. You're just not going to drive a school bus into a garage made for a sedan.

There are hundreds of ways you can ad lib during sexual exploration and the only limit to what you and your partner can do is your imagination.

29. Play a Guessing Game

One fun thing to do to help spark the sexual fires between you and your lover is playing a guessing game. On your own, start by laying out a variety of items that could be used in sensual ways on the bed or nightstand. You may want to try the following items:

- Feathers.
- Ties.
- A hairbrush.
- Frozen foods.
- Candlesticks (put a condom on one and go to town, or light them up and—carefully—drip the hot wax onto your partner's body).
- Electric toothbrush (not the business end though please).
- Cell phone (put it on vibrate and watch your partner squirm).
- Ice cubes.

After you have arranged your items, blindfold your partner and lead him into bed. Pick up each item and find a tantalizing way to use it on his body and ask him to guess what each object is as you do. For each right answer, you can reward him and for each wrong answer, he can reward you. Playing games in bed with your lover can inject some lightheartedness into your sex life and, when life is stressful, can be an effective way to relax and get back to having amazing sex.

30. *Your Marriage Is More Important Than Your Kids*

Here's a little secret: You don't have to spend all of your free time with your kids. Of course, we're not suggesting that you ditch them completely if they're making you crazy, but a little alone time away with your partner is one key to having a happy marriage in which you and he feel emotionally connected. And part of that emotional connection stems from a fulfilling sex life.

HE **SAYS** . . .

Some couples spend all their time together worrying about and working hard to get to the relaxing wonderful times when they'll get to truly enjoy their time together. Well, those supposedly wonderful times when you *may* be happy together may never come. And *if* they ever do, you'll kick yourself for not seizing the moments before. Guess what: All we have in the world is *this* very moment. More good times may or may not come. Enjoy this moment, live it to the fullest, as if it were your last. That is something you're very unlikely to ever regret.

Think of a happy marriage as a positive cycle. The more you work to enjoy sex and other intimate moments with your partner, the more loving you two will likely be to your children. When you're unhappy, fighting with your partner, and feeling emotionally divorced, it can take a real toll on your health, your relationships with others, and your self-esteem. It causes your children stress, and, in turn, they may start acting out. But, when you nurture a supportive, happy, sexually fulfilling relationship with your partner, you create a positive atmosphere within the home. Your children will be happier and less worried about whether or not their parents love each other and you'll probably experience less strife between you and them (and your positive role modeling may even help them later in their own relationships as they will have exposure to a relationship worth emulating). As a result, you'll be happier because you're not fighting with your kids and that will give you the emotional energy to have fun with your partner. This results in more great sex.

HE **SAYS . . .**

So many people grew up in families where the parents didn't really love each other in a romantic sense, if at all. And many people grew up thinking that marriage is horrible, and that it means being sentenced to be with a person who makes you unhappy. Don't do this to your children. Show them what a loving family can mean. Love the person you're with and, if you can't, then choose to be with someone you can love.

Honestly, getting a babysitter once a week so that you and your partner can go out on a nice, intimate, romantic date doesn't make you a bad parent. Sending the kids to their grandparents' house for the night so you can get it on in the living room does not make you a bad parent. Taking a vacation, just the two of you, does not make you a bad parent. Closing the bedroom door for some grownup time does not make you a bad parent. But these things are absolutely necessary to keep the spark alive in your marriage. Letting your sex life die along with your marriage sets the wrong example for your kids. Be a good parent by showing your children what a loving, intimate, and happy relationship looks like. They will follow your example into their own adult lives.

31. *A Trench Coat Is Always in Style*

It can be freeing—and seductive—to face your fears and let go of inhibitions. So, take it to the next level and go on your next date wearing absolutely nothing but a long coat. It's not illegal or immoral, but it sure is sexy! Trust us, your man will love the fact that your jacket is the only thing between him and your beautiful body. By the end of the night, he won't want to wait to slip that jacket off your shoulders and slide you between the sheets. If you're really feeling free spirited—or your man can't control himself on the ride home—you can loosen the coat in the car for a little spontaneous fondling.

32. *You Can Get Off without Letting Him In*

Are you really surprised? Of course you can get off with *or* without intercourse. It's very possible and healthy for a woman to orgasm in multiple ways—and multiple times—through penetration, masturbation (alone or with a partner), or with the help of sex toys. Just remember that masturbation and intercourse are very different experiences. Masturbation does not diminish the experience of sex and sex toys do not replace intercourse. They are all fun and exciting ways to help you reach your peak.

*Sex*MYTH: **If You Can't Orgasm Through Intercourse, Something Is Wrong with You** Less than 70 percent of women can achieve orgasm through intercourse alone. So don't be afraid, or embarrassed, to reach down and touch your clitoris during sex. It'll greatly increase your chances of orgasm and will increase his excitement level at the same time. Also, don't be afraid to ask him to wait for you to orgasm. Simultaneous orgasm doesn't just magically happen in real life the way it does in romance novels. It requires communication between you and your partner during sex.

Is one kind of orgasm better than the other? No, but an interesting point to ponder is that many women claim that orgasms are more intense through masturbation. If you've been there, you know what we're talking about. If not, here's why: While you may feel emotional closeness and fullness from your partner being inside of you, you may not experience the same intensity that you do with a masturbation-induced orgasm. When you realize that the vaginal walls contain relatively few nerve endings, this starts to make more sense. Add to this the fact that you're more likely to stimulate your clitoris, which is highly sensitive and full of nerve endings, during masturbation, it's no wonder that a little self-love feels more intense. Plus, you know when, where, and how to touch yourself because the feedback is built in. When having sex with a partner, you have to give feedback and assume that he knows how to respond, etc.

HE **SAYS . . .**

Hollywood always shows couples having hot, sweaty, incredible sex and climaxing at the exact same moment—after which they both pass out together. Yeah. That only happens in the movies and ever-so-rarely in real life. Don't worry about it though; just remember your partner after your own climax—or make sure your partner remembers you after his.

To have stronger orgasms with your partner, feedback is critical. So the next time you two are getting hot and heavy, ask him to touch, rub, caress, and/or press your clitoris with his fingers (and tell him or show him how you like it). Or better yet, do it yourself with your fingers or a vibrator. It can be a real turn-on for him to watch you pleasure yourself.

33. *The Female Libido Does Exist*

The female libido is a touchy subject, and sometimes women don't even know what it is. Is it the same as a sex drive? How does it function? How do you know if you have a high or a low libido? Here are the answers to these questions and to the ones you didn't even think to ask!

*Sex*MYTH: **Men Are Always Ready for Sex** Though most ads and men's magazines will have you believing otherwise, this just simply isn't true. A man's sex drive is subject to some of the same things that can derail a woman's—relationship issues, stress, lack of sleep, depression, etc.—so if he hasn't been interested lately, don't think he's no longer attracted to you. Instead, sit down with him and check in with his inner feelings. He might really appreciate being able to get some stressors off his chest.

What Is the Female Libido?

Libido refers to a person's sex drive, and both men and women have a libido. Not surprisingly, the typical male libido is quite different from the typical female libido! (What isn't different about men and women?) In fact, the only thing that is similar about a female libido and a male libido is that both men and women can have high, moderate, or low libidos. Typically, a man's libido is highest when he's in his late teens and early twenties, while a woman's libido is highest when she gets a little older, typically early thirties to forties. If you don't fit inside this box though, don't worry. Everyone is different!

Is My Libido Too Low?

Lots of things can affect a woman's libido—everything from outside factors such as stress, emotional issues, and even childhood issues, to medications and exercise. A change in your libido can be surprising. You may not have had much sexual desire before, but now suddenly find yourself interested in sex at every turn, or you may experience a lowering in your libido where you used to crave sex a fair amount of the time and now you feel disinterested. If you feel your libido is low, take a look at the factors in your life that could be having an effect. Are you on any medications that could lower your sex drive? Are you eating, sleeping, and exercising enough? Are you going through tough emotional times? All of these factors are possible culprits, and you might find that a combination of them is wreaking havoc on your sex life. Here are some proven libido boosters that you can implement right away:

- **Touch:** Many times a low libido is caused simply by a lack of affection and casual touch in nonsexual situations. Hugging, holding hands, or getting a massage without the expectation of sex all have the interesting effect of increasing a woman's sex drive.

- **Yoga or Tantra:** Yoga and tantra can have the effect of bringing you and your partner into sync emotionally as a couple. Being emotionally in sync is critical for libido in both partners.

- **Quality Time:** Spend time together just doing nothing. Enjoy some casual conversation. Take a long walk. Our lives can be so hectic these days that we even forget to stop and breathe—no wonder we're not interested in sex. Set a goal to spend at least fifteen minutes per day, just the two of you, for thirty days and see what a difference it makes.

- **Better Sex:** One of the biggest reasons for not wanting to have sex is boring and unfulfilling sex. Make sure that you and your partner are truly satisfying each other. Talk about what you do and don't like and try new things often. Don't get stuck in a rut!
- **Eat Healthy:** There is an old saying that claims we are what we eat and, in regard to libido, foods that taste good but make you feel lazy and lifeless afterward will definitely not get you in the mood. So eat something energizing that makes you want to get up and at 'em in the bedroom.
- **Supplements:** Sometimes, a woman's body needs more than what she can get from food. This is where supplements come in. Taking a high-quality, natural supplement such as iron, folic acid, calcium, vitamin D, ginseng, black cohosh, chasteberry, l-arginine, ginkgo, or yohimbe, can help to fill in the gaps in your diet and help you prepare for passion.

34. He Wants You to Want Him

In many cultures, even today, men are expected to be macho, to suck it up, and to never cry or show emotion. Women are often still taught to be passive, nonaggressive, and a tender influence in their relationships. On top of that, until recently, women were not taught how to enjoy, much less initiate, sex. It was simply an obligation to be fulfilled in their marriages. Men were supposed to know what to do, when to do it, and how to do it.

Ugh!

Taking charge in the bedroom can be a terrifying thought for many women. You may be quite comfortable playing a submissive role in the bedroom and have no desire to change. But, most likely, your man will love it if you initiate sex—and he will show his appreciation in the bedroom. As you know, your partner is not a mind reader and he only knows what you want if you ask for it. So, how do you bring your sexuality more into balance so that both you and your partner can enjoy the experience?

HE **SAYS** . . .

Ladies, don't underestimate the power of feedback! As a guy, I can tell you that there are times when we're not quite sure where to go or what to do. Tell us what you want, and we'll be more than happy to oblige.

As a woman, you have to become comfortable with your sexuality and learn to ask for what you need and desire in a positive and loving manner. Your partner should not be the only one asking for sex; don't be afraid to be forceful in the bedroom—he'll love it! Learn to express yourself sexually and take charge.

Taking charge can mean many different things, from simply asking for sex to putting on the most hard-core dominatrix show. What you decide to do depends on your level of comfort in the relationship, your own sexuality, and what you truly want. We challenge you to push these boundaries on a daily basis. To get you started, here are ten quick ways that you can take charge in the bedroom:

1. Send him a text message telling him that you're in the bedroom naked and horny.
2. Join him in the shower when he's getting ready for work.
3. Whisper in his ear "I need you. Right now!" and lead him to the bedroom.
4. The next time you have sex, be on top.

5. Give him a blow job while he's watching TV.
6. Put a blindfold on him or tie his hands behind his back while you have your way with him.
7. Tell him what you want in the bedroom and describe how it feels—in detail.
8. Have him be your sex slave for the day.
9. Send him on a sexual scavenger hunt.
10. Wake him up at night with a sexy surprise.

35. Position Yourself for Pleasure: Try the Lotus

The Lotus position is an all-time favorite; it's incredibly intimate, but also provides a terrific penetration angle. In fact, this is quite possibly the most intimate sexual position there is! If you're the type of woman who wants intimacy and ecstasy, this position will give you both at the same time. Not only are you face to face with your partner, but your bodies are totally entwined together. This is a great position to reconnect, even fully clothed.

To get into the Lotus position, your partner should sit cross-legged and you should sit on his lap, facing him. You and your partner should then wrap your arms and legs around each other in a very intimate hug and begin rocking back and forth. Before long, you'll be gazing into his eyes and screaming his name.

36. Don't Be Critical

If you really want to crush a man's interest in sex, feel free to criticize him or make him feel inadequate. This doesn't mean that you shouldn't be confident, voice your sexual needs, or feel comfortable telling him that you prefer he move a little to the left, but men take great pride in their ability to be studs in the bedroom. So, if he is not living up to his passion potential, you need to tread very carefully. Coming right out and telling your partner that he isn't fulfilling your needs is a recipe for disaster. For every 100 things you tell a man he does right, it only takes one criticism to erase all the hard work. Yes, this sensitivity can be annoying, but here are five tips to help you critique without criticizing:

1. Tell him what he's doing right rather than what he's doing wrong.
2. Gently guide his hands or other body parts into a position that feels good and then tell him what he's doing right.
3. Demonstrate for him how to do it the way you like it and then tell him what he's doing right.
4. Gently suggest that you'd like to try something new and then tell him what he's doing right.
5. If you must tell him that he's doing something wrong, tell him in a way that makes it about the action, not in a way that makes it his fault—and then tell him what he's doing right.

HE **SAYS . . .**

The idea that every man magically knows exactly how to please a woman in bed is ludicrous. You don't expect us to know how to play the piano or drive a forklift—or most anything else frankly—without learning first, but somehow we're just supposed to inherently know how to please a woman. It sounds totally silly, but our culture puts great importance on a man just knowing, and, oftentimes, we're afraid to bust that. So, ladies, be aware of that fact, cut us some slack, and let us know what we can do better next time.

When you approach him using one of these five tactics, you'll be that much closer to achieving the best sex of your life—and you'll also be less likely to end up with a sulking lover, which is never a turn-on.

37. It's Okay to Do It During That Time of the Month

People check in with us on this issue all the time and our immediate reaction to this question is always "Why are you asking us instead of your partner?" This is something that should be discussed with your lover as each person's sexual preferences and needs are different. If you're comfortable with the idea of having sex or messing around during your period, then ask your partner what his opinion is, or the next time you're on your period and he tries to make a move, just let him know and see how he responds. If he doesn't seem to care, you'll have your answer.

However, it's important to keep in mind that first and foremost, the option of having sex during your period has an awful lot to do with how you personally feel about it. Are you the type who experiences mood swings or has to deal with horrible cramping? Are you normally withdrawn during this particular time of the month? These are all very legitimate reasons to avoid sex during your period.

Ironically, sex can potentially alleviate some of the discomfort that menstruation presents for a woman. Sex promotes blood flow which has the potential to minimize headaches and even relax cramping, and that's not saying anything about the obvious tension release! Thanks to endorphins released when you get down, sex can also be a great kick-start to feeling re-energized during a downswing of your mood. This can also be a time where the surge of hormones can create a heightened sense of libido, which can certainly benefit sexual activity.

*Sex*MYTH: **You Can't Get Pregnant on Your Period** Wrong! You can get pregnant anytime: Before your period, on your period, and after your period. Sperm can stay in the vagina for up to seven days, so even if you're shedding the last egg, the sperm might still be in there when you release the next one. So, unless you want to get pregnant—and maybe you do—it's important to use protection or hormonal birth control.

Also, we should let you know that period-sex really isn't all that different than sex any other time. Sure it can be a little messier—and wetter—than usual, but sometimes that just adds to the kink! So, even if you're not sure that you're comfortable with sex during this time of the month, an attempt couldn't hurt. If it's not for you, then at least you know. But if it does work then you can enjoy a whole new experience going forward.

What If My Guy Doesn't Like It?

Now if it's your guy who would rather avoid the dirty lovin' at this time of month, well, that's a whole other situation. For many guys a woman's time of month is a turn-off. This is mainly a mental reaction because physically things aren't all that different. If this is something you want to try, but your partner is hesitant because of the blood, why not turn off the lights? If all goes according to plan, once you two are turned on and ready to go, his focus will likely be on how things *feel* versus how they may look. If your partner prefers a little less clean up (not to mention the obvious protection from risk), you two can always choose to use a condom. Also, get yourself a large towel to spread over the bed sheets and off you go!

Going Oral

So, if you are into the idea of having sex while you have your period and you and your partner have both moved beyond any hesitations then we can take things to the next level: oral sex. You'll find that even men who don't take issue with period sex, draw the line with oral sex during that time of the month. But again, everything regarding intimacy and comfort level is based on personal choice.

However, what many men don't consider when it comes to period sex is that flow levels vary throughout your time. Sure there will be heavier days where you can expect a little more fluid but there are also lighter days which might be a good time to venture into making an attempt.

Oral sex during your period can stay focused on the clitoris, which is mainly away from the flow and won't be quite as shocking to your man. If you are on your back there is also less potential for mess. Your partner can also use oral dams (like a condom for their mouths during oral sex) at this time of month. In return, if you are not comfortable with giving him oral sex after he's gotten messy, put a condom on him (a fresh one) before going down.

38. *Sleep* Au Naturel

Sleeping naked has many rewards. Not the least of which is that it makes sex a lot more likely to happen. So what are some of the advantages of sleeping naked with your partner?

Releases Oxytocin

Oxytocin is a hormone released with skin-to-skin contact. Touching skin-to-skin and head-to-toe all night long will provide you with a steady stream of this beneficial hormone. Some of the benefits of oxytocin include an increased sense of well-being, decreased heart rate, reduction of stress hormones, increased sense of trust, and—*drum roll please!*—sexual arousal!

Puts You in the Mood

Getting into the mood for sex can be a challenge for many women. We tend to stay in our heads and worry about being tired, or that the kids will hear, or whatever we are stressing about that day. Instead of putting you in the mood for sexual contact, this type of worry, in fact, tends to make you feel alone and isolated. Many women will simply answer "Not tonight, dear" if their man initiates sex just because they have too much going on in their heads. Slipping under the sheets in your birthday suit stimulates sexual feelings no matter who you are or what is going on in your head.

HE SAYS . . .

Guess what, ladies? Seeing you go to bed naked is very erotic for us. It sends an invitation. Shows us you're interested. Yes, please!

Creates Desire

One of the main reasons that women don't feel like sex is a sense of disconnect between the couple. When you feel disconnected from your partner, you may lose a sense of desire for him. Sleeping nude helps to break down those barriers.

Sleeping skin-to-skin can also increase your sense of bonding. Think about it, when you first started dating you couldn't keep your hands off each other, right? The more you touch, the closer you feel to your partner . . . and increased bonding equals more sex!

Having more sex has many health benefits and increases the chances of your marriage lasting. Okay, I am not talking marathon sex here. I am also not talking having sex five times a day. In fact, even once or twice a day can do wonders. By spending half an hour a day in the most enjoyable and healthy exercise you can partake in, you will live longer, feel more satisfied with your life, and be healthier. Not to mention it will increase the odds of your marriage living as long as you do!

So, slip in between those sheets in the buff and enjoy all the benefits—over and over and over again!

39. *Men Love Foreplay, Too*

Here's something you may not know: Guys enjoy foreplay just as much as women. The type of foreplay your partner wants is just a little different than what you're interested in. So what is your man looking for? Well, all men love a good strip tease. While women may not consider strip teases foreplay, men love them! Come on! You didn't think women were the only ones who love to be teased, did you?

And here's another big surprise. Most men don't want strange women giving them a lap dance. Your man would prefer to see you do it for him. But here's the thing, many women are too shy or self-conscious to strip for their men because they are thinking about their flaws. But all he sees is a really sexy, beautiful woman. Trust me on this!

You should be the one stripping for your man, so get over those insecurities. You don't have to slide upside-down down a metal pole to turn him on. Here are some basic strip tease moves that are guaranteed to have him putting dollars in your thong!

*Sex*MYTH: **Men Don't Like Foreplay** Men love foreplay—it just may not be the same kind of foreplay that you like. Men are very visual and love to be teased. Seeing you in a sexy dress or lingerie or receiving a text telling him what you're going to do later, can send your man into single-minded thinking about having sex with you.

The Setup

You'll want to dress in layers because you're going to be taking things off very gradually. Also, opt for sheer and clingy fabrics that accentuate your feminine curves. Place a chair for him in the middle of the room so you can easily move all the way around him. Put a second chair, stool, or ottoman nearby for you to use. Playing some music with a good strong sexy beat in the background is a good idea and if you're really nervous feel free to have a pre-dance cocktail. Just don't drink too much because you might be too clumsy to dance! If you really want to spice things up, you can add a no-touch, no-talk rule, or better yet, tie his hands behind his back.

Doing the Dance

Just forget about how silly you feel and relax. Remember, all he sees is an incredible sensuous woman. By the way, you don't actually have to dance. Move in a way that feels natural to you.

Here are some basic moves that will drive him wild:

- Move around him slowly.
- Move your hands slowly over your body.
- Move your hands over his body—but only briefly.
- Bend over so he can see down your shirt.
- Bend over so that he can get a peek at your bottom.
- Straddle one of his legs and lower yourself onto it, then briefly rub your crotch against his leg.
- Brush his face with your breasts.
- Whisper in his ear from behind—give him hints of what's to come.
- Use a chair or stool to lean on, straddle, bend over, etc.
- Here's the big one—make direct eye contact with him.

HE **SAYS . . .**

Not all men want to go to strip clubs and watch strange women undress. If you have a truly open, trusting, and sexually liberated relationship with your man, he's unlikely to want to see some woman take her clothes off. For me, paying to see women undress is not that different than paying to have sex with someone, and both are (for me, personally) quite unappealing. Strip clubs hold great mystique for young guys who just need to see breasts, but for a man who thinks his woman is the sexiest ever, watching some girl prance around naked for money is just not a turn-on. So, instead of hassling your man about going to a strip club, consider taking away his desire for the strip club by fulfilling his fantasies.

Getting Naked

The key thing to remember here is to take your time. Actually getting naked should take several minutes. Remember, the idea here is to tease him and leave him begging for more. Slide an article of clothing aside, showing some skin for just a moment, and then hide it again. Remember, he likes seeing you touch the parts of you that he wants to touch, so stroking, squeezing, and rubbing your breasts and crotch is a good idea both with and without clothes.

Don't forget to actually have fun and make good eye contact, letting him know that you're enjoying yourself.

The Happy Ending

Your man will be extremely aroused when you're finished, so if you decide to have sex afterward, don't expect him to last very long. One way to draw out the pleasure a little longer and to ensure that you're not left hanging is to get into the Lap Dance position, but instead of letting him control the thrusting, masturbate while gently moving on him. It's up to you how to end this, but your man will certainly enjoy it if you give him an orgasm right there in the chair—or on the floor, or in the bedroom, or anywhere else for that matter. But remember, it's not about finishing at the same time, but rather about making sure both of you make it to the finish line!

40. You Can Learn to Love Oral Sex

You know how to give great head, but now it's time to learn how to love receiving oral sex. This is a big problem for many women. You see, women tend to want to control their orgasms, which is a huge mistake. Here are some tips to help you become a better receiver:

Relax

A woman has to be completely relaxed to have an orgasm. If your mind is on your job, if you're self-conscious about how your body looks, if you're trying to have an orgasm, etc., you're not going to be relaxed. Instead, you'll be tense, and your body won't allow you to release an orgasm—or even enjoy what your partner is doing to you down there. So your biggest job is to just simply relax. Here are three simple ways to relax and unwind:

1. **Love Your Environment:** Create a relaxing environment in your bedroom and bathroom so, when you get home, you'll be able to take a few minutes to yourself to unwind and relax. When you come home from a busy day, make sure your partner knows you love him and that you're happy to see him—and then politely excuse yourself for thirty minutes of me-time. Relax, read, meditate, or take a short nap so that you can shift gears from busy time to romantic time.

2. **Turn on the Shower (or Bath):** Invite your partner to take a shower or bath with you. We prefer a shower because baths can sometimes be too relaxing, but do whatever you like best. This is not the time for intense sexual activity, but rather a time for creating intimacy and closeness. Wash your partner's hair, wash your partner's body, and just be close to him. Another added benefit of taking a shower or bath together is that you'll both be clean and smell nice

when you're done. It can be hard to relax during oral sex if you know you need to clean up.

3. **Try Massage.** The last step to help you get in the mood for sex is a massage. This is not intended to be a deep tissue massage, but rather a slow sensual massage. Use a good massage cream or oil. If your man doesn't like to give massages, simply ask him if he'll rub lotion on your body in long sweeping strokes. If you're lying on the bed naked with a bottle of lotion in your hands, it's doubtful that he'll refuse.

HE **SAYS . . .**

Cleanliness absolutely matters. One of the things guys really like about women is that they always smell nice and clean! Even after a long day, getting cleaned up for intimate time goes a long way and makes your man feel special. Maybe even special enough to get himself cleaned up too!

Communicate

After all, how can you expect your man to know what you like if you can't tell him, or show him? Verbal communication is best so that you can tell him exactly what you like and how you like it, but simple moans at the right time and subtle movement of your hips will let him know that you're enjoying what he's doing.

Lend a Hand

If you're worried that you won't get off with just oral stimulation, take things into your own hands. Don't be afraid to reach down and stimulate your clitoris while he's giving you oral sex, or even ask him to do it for you. It's very common for a woman to want or need multiple types of stimulation to reach orgasm. So don't stress out about it. There's no need for that—if you enjoy having orgasms and that's what it takes, then so be it! Just relax and have fun.

Just Let Go

If you think your man can't get you off during oral sex, then you won't get off. But, if you follow our suggestions above, you'll be arching your back in ecstasy in no time. Remember, if you can orgasm by yourself, you can orgasm with your partner. During oral sex, he may be in the driver's seat, but you're the navigator. Relax, know what you like—and fill him in—and feel free to help get yourself there. Oral sex can be great, so really let go and give it a try. You'll have better and more frequent orgasms and his confidence will grow with each success.

HE **SAYS . . .**

From a man's perspective, it's actually quite nice to see a woman fully engaged enough in sex play and comfortable enough to help stimulate herself by lending a helping hand, etc. It makes it feel like she's more in the game too, as opposed to just being the spectator you're working on.

41. *Your Man Will Thank You for Doing Those Kegels*

One of the reasons why some women have a hard time having an orgasm is because of weak pelvic floor muscles. These are the muscles that surround the vaginal opening, and are the same muscles a woman uses to hold in her urine. When a woman has an orgasm the PC muscles spasm, which means that strong PC muscles mean stronger and longer lasting orgasms! You can develop these muscles by doing Kegel exercises for as little as five minutes, three times a day. Here are a few exercises that will give you a feel of what it's like to squeeze your PC muscles:

- Every time you go to the bathroom to pee, try to stop the flow of urine when you are sitting on the toilet. If you can do it, you are using the right muscles. Urinate, stop, urinate again, stop, and repeat.
- Get comfortable lying on your bed and insert a finger in your vagina. Try to squeeze the muscles as hard as you can and then release. You should feel your vaginal walls clamping down on your finger when you've got it right.
- If you really want to give these muscles a workout, you can even buy different levels of vaginal weights from your favorite sex-toy store.

*Sex*MYTH: **Men Want Sex More Than Women** We beg to differ. Women want sex just as much as men. It just takes a little more effort to get a girl warmed up and she tends to be easily distracted by the worries of the day. In addition, hormone fluctuations cause women to want sex more during certain times of the month. All of this definitely does not mean that women don't want sex as much as men, only that it may take a little more encouragement for women to remember that they want it.

And once you get the hang of squeezing your PC muscles, you can do it discreetly just about anywhere—sitting in traffic, standing in line, even while watching television. Just a quick note: Make sure that you're only squeezing these muscles and not your stomach or bottom. And don't forget to breathe.

42. Knowledge Is Power—Especially When We're Talking about Orgasms

Have you ever heard of the Four Phases of Female Orgasm? No? Well, it's high time you did. These four phases were introduced in the original sexual response cycle (defined by Masters and Johnson in 1966) and describe the process women go through on the way to sexual bliss. While this is all great in theory, recognize that women are all different and may not each experience orgasm in this order or in this way. It's quite possible to move between phases, back and forth between different levels of excitement. Here is a quick summary of Masters and Johnson's response cycle.

1. **Excitement Phase:** In this phase, you respond to sexual stimuli and you begin to get wet. Here's the thing that's not discussed in the study: Sexual stimuli can mean many different things to many different people; it basically refers to whatever gets you aroused.

2. **Plateau Phase:** This phase represents the time between the initial arousal and excitement, up until you actually reach orgasm. This is where most women get stuck. (Forget about what you have to do at work tomorrow . . . we're serious!) Stop thinking and focus on just letting go.

3. **Orgasm Phase:** You know what this phase feels like, ladies! Different women feel orgasms differently—intense contractions, physical shaking, increased heart rate, warming or flushing of the skin, feeling like you have to urinate, the list goes on and on. The common thread is that it's a feeling of release. This phase may also consist of muscle contractions around the vagina, uterus, and anus.

4. **Resolution Phase:** This phase is the period of time immediately following an orgasm, when the body begins to return to its normal state. An important note on this one is that it's very possible for women to jump back to the beginning and experience multiple orgasms. To do this, some women require a longer resolution phase, but others can jump right back into the excitement phase almost immediately.

HE **SAYS . . .**

Many women can experience multiple orgasms straight out of the box. That is totally not fair. We want to get back in the game without a break too (which experts say is possible, but they also say Bigfoot has been spotted again), but more often than not, we'll need a nap first.

43. *Intimacy and Desire Go Hand in Hand*

It happens all the time: Two people fall in love, have sex like rabbits, and become comfortable with each other. And then, although they love their relationship, it starts to dawn on them that their sex life has stagnated. What went wrong? Why does this happen? In the beginning of a relationship, our bodies are pumping out love chemicals—such as oxytocin—that cause both bonding and sexual attraction. As those bonds are formed and the body becomes more used to your new partner, the chemicals start to drop off. So, what are you to do? To get back to having the best sex of your life, let's consider the differences between the two of you. Having a deeper understanding of your partner makes it easier to empathize with him and this stronger connection makes it easier to feel more sexually free.

Men and Women

When women are in relationships, their sexual desire for their partners often stems from feeling close, emotional bonds with them. If women feel the levels of intimacy are high, they're more likely to want to have sex. On the other hand, simply having a physical attraction to their partners—whether they're in relationships or just dating around—can arouse most men. Not surprisingly, this can create a wee bit of conflict. Think about it: Have you ever been in a position where your partner is trying to fondle you and you get annoyed because you'd rather be seduced than groped? Does this happen more when you haven't been having sex in a little while? Though you don't have to respond in kind and immediately hop into bed with him, consider that your partner is not trying to treat you like a sex object. Instead, he is making an effort to be intimate by showing you he is physically attracted to you and interested in making love. Realizing he is trying to help your relationship may help you to be less annoyed and less dismissive of his advances. So, if you want to improve your sex life—and we know you do—don't just brush him off.

Redirecting the Ship

Sometimes, guys just don't get the picture. If he's still driving you mad by randomly squeezing your nipples or doing some other obnoxious behavior and you haven't had any luck by trying to subtly show him what you *do* like, feel free to let him know what you are looking for. Your man will likely respond much better to that than you telling him what he's doing wrong. When he feels he's wrong, he will tend to sulk and be less flirtatious, less touchy feely, and less interested in sex. And that's not what either of you want.

HE **SAYS . . .**

Look ladies. If you're naked, we'll do whatever you want us to. After all, who can refuse a hot, naked girl on the bed saying, "Would you rub some of this on my back?" No guy that I can think of.

Communication is the key to a healthy relationship but communicating with positive language and actions usually results in the best outcomes. Men love to please (especially when there's something in it for them), so make it a point to show him what really turns you on. Instead of giving attention to the things that drive you nuts, pay extra-special attention to what he does that you like. The more you praise something, the more often he's likely to do it. So, instead of getting angry at him the next time he squeezes your nipple (though, to be honest, we'd be hard-pressed not to get a little aggravated ourselves), try to be nicer about it. Raise your eyebrow, take his hand off your breast and guide it to somewhere you want it to be, and tell him how good that feels. He'll quickly get the picture and you'll end up having much more and much better sex.

44. *Viagra Isn't the Only Miracle Pill*
If you want to boost your libido, there are supplements and medications called *female libido enhancers* that can help you enjoy a

more natural and healthy sex life. Some libido enhancers are herbal formulas, others are pills, and still others are put directly on the vagina. Normally, a combination of both pills and external creams or gels has been reported to provide the best results.

Before taking any supplement or libido enhancer, check with your doctor or qualified herbalist. Not all supplements will affect everyone in the same way. Here are just a few of the nonprescription libido enhancers available:

- **St. John's Wort:** Known as a mood enhancer, it may also lift your libido. Just keep in mind it can also affect the effectiveness of oral contraceptives.
- **Korean Gingseng:** Gingseng is known as an energy booster and stress reliever so it may also help increase your libido—especially if its lowered level is related to stress issues.
- **Ginkgo Biloba:** Ginkgo is known for increasing focus and blood flow, so you get the idea.
- **Vibrance Cream:** This is a cream claiming to boost a woman's libido within minutes.
- **Zestra Feminine Arousal Fluid:** This is an oil claiming to increase arousal in women when applied during foreplay.

There are many other nonprescription alternatives out there to help you increase your libido, but you should always do your research before trying any of these products. Know the ingredients, disclaimers, and all possible side effects before putting anything in or on your body.

45. *Three Can Be Great Company in the Bedroom*

For some couples, it can be quite arousing to bring a third party into the bedroom. The novelty of being with another person combined with seeing how your partner reacts with another person and with watching you touch another person can be exhilarating. Also, you'll get to enjoy the chance to be pleasured by two people at once, which can lead to some really interesting sensations.

*Sex*MYTH: **Fantasizing about Women Means I'm a Lesbian**

It's perfectly acceptable to fantasize about whatever you want. If you find yourself fantasizing about women, it doesn't necessarily mean you're a lesbian, but just that you find women attractive. They are, of course, otherwise so many artists wouldn't have painted and sculpted them throughout the ages. And, if you do find yourself wanting to explore having sexual relations with women, that's absolutely okay too. Be open to your sexuality. As long as it involves consenting adults, there's nothing wrong with whatever turns you on.

The Rules

In order for both you and your partner to enjoy the threesome experience to the fullest and to make sure it ends up with both of you having amazing sex and not in an amazing fight, it's important to lay out the ground rules *ahead* of time. Be sure to ask yourself the following questions:

- What is permitted?
- What is off limits?

- Will the third person stay the night or leave afterward?
- Will all three of you join in or will one of you watch while the other two engage in sexual activity?

Also, be sure to discuss any concerns or reservations you have about bringing a third person into the bedroom and make sure all of these concerns are fully addressed before going out into the field, so to speak. And, after the experience, it's important to talk again with your partner to make sure no one has any lasting jealousy or other issues that could affect your relationship.

Finding the Right Person

The right person makes all the difference in a threesome. Ask yourself the following questions when figuring out what you and your partner are looking for:

- Do you want a male or female?
- Are you comfortable sharing someone as fit or fitter than you?
- Do you want to introduce a stranger into your dynamic or a free-spirited friend?
- Are you interested in someone in a particular age range?

When approaching the third person to see if they're interested, it's important to avoid coming off as creepy. Just be straightforward and refrain from pressuring them. There's no telling whether they'll be flattered or appalled, but if you're cordial, you certainly have a better chance.

Play It Safe!

When having sex with a third, possibly unknown person, it is extremely important that both you and your partner use protection. This way, you can focus on having fun—and enjoying the amazingly kinky sex—and not on whether you'll catch something.

46. Lube Is a Girl's Best Friend

There happen to be hundreds of different types of lubricants out there. Some are made specifically for sexual use and others happen to work well for sex, but might also be good on a slice of bread. Here's the down and dirty on what you need to know about lube, including:

- What should not be used as lube?
- What kind of lube should you get?
- What can you use it for and why?

Do I Need Lube?

In short, yes! It can help reduce friction, help keep a condom on and safe, and help heighten both your and your partner's pleasure. Have a good bottle of your favorite lubricant ready and you're bound to have a more enjoyable experience.

Don't be afraid to experiment with different types of lubricants, including lubes with different consistencies, different textures, different flavors, and different additives. There are numbing lubricants—which should never be used for anal sex—and even lubricants that can increase sensitivity and heighten pleasure. There are many different types of lubricants available online, including lubes in convenient pump dispensers for mess-free fun.

What Is Not Lube?

Lotion isn't lube (unless you're giving a genital massage), and neither is saliva (unless you're giving or receiving a blow job), or even just plain water. While you might be tempted to just use something you have around the house in the heat of the moment, you're much better off if you plan ahead and get yourself a good lubricant that will work well for what you need.

Oil-based lubricants can work well for men during masturbation or massage, but oil-based lubricants are bad news for women during sex and even during masturbation. Oil breeds bacteria very easily and keeps it there—it is very difficult to wash off.

If you're choosing a lubricant to use for sex, use the ones made specifically for sex! You'll find that almost all of them are water-based lubricants.

Water-Based Lubricant

Water-based lubricant is by far the most popular lube on the market. Why is water-based lubricant so popular? First of all, this type of lube doesn't break down condoms. That's the most important factor—oil-based lubricants can weaken latex condoms and make them nearly useless. Unless you want babies or sexually transmitted diseases, you're better off using a good, water-based lubricant. Secondly, it's sold almost everywhere—even your local grocery store sells water-based lube! The other bonuses that come with water-based lube is that it washes off easily and it doesn't stain sheets or clothing!

Silicone-Based Lubricants

Silicone-based lubricants are great for those who have glycerin allergies, or for those who want to use lubrication under water such as in the shower or hot tub. Silicone-based lube won't break down a condom, but it also won't wash away in the same way that a water-based lubricant will. The only downside? Like oil-based lubricants, it's difficult to get off afterward.

47. Sometimes, Kinky Isn't Better

Once you start playing around with the kinkier side of sex, it's easy to get caught up in trying out new sex positions all the time, enhancing your tantra skills, or just tying each other up. But sometimes, it's important to let go of trying to keep up with the Joneses. Sometimes, it's important to just have—and want—simple, plain, ordinary, missionary position sex. Nothing fancy. Just you and your partner connecting and sharing in your intimate experience.

*Sex*MYTH: **Happy Couples Do It All the Time** You know what is going to kill your sex life? Holding it up to the same standard as another couple's. If your friend says she and her boyfriend have sex three times a day, be happy for her, but that doesn't mean just because you have sex twice a week your sex life is bad. All that matters is that you and your partner are happy in the relationship and both sexually satisfied. Of course, if you find yourself wanting more, initiate it!

First Time

When it's your first time with a particular partner, it's probably best to not go overboard with the kink, unless you met them in say, a dungeon. Allow yourselves to explore each other and get to know what turns each other on (and off) before adding anything else to the mix. This way, when props just aren't available you'll still be able to have great sex.

Prop-Free

If your sex life usually involves props, here's a tip: Schedule a prop-free sex session. By doing so, it will allow you and your partner to reconnect on a deep level when it's just the two of you and you aren't distracted by how fun your new toy is. Over time, your tastes may have changed and this is a great way to reacquaint yourself with what arouses your partner and for your partner to do the same with you.

48. Position Yourself for Pleasure: Try the Bridge

Are you ready for this? This is an advanced position that is not for the weak. It's both a workout and sexual position. With the Bridge position, you need to be facing upward, using all four limbs to hold your body weight off the bed or floor. If you need to cheat a little, use an ottoman or the arm of a cushy sofa. The advantage of the Bridge position is that you are elevated, which will give him a better angle of penetration to stimulate your G-spot, sort of like a flipped over Doggie style. And because you're not laying flat on the bed, he can pull you toward him and thrust harder for longer— assuming that your arms and legs can hold up! While this position takes a little more practice and stamina than some of the other positions, once you get there, it'll be another favorite, especially if you like to play hard.

49. *Anal Sex Can Actually Be Amazing*

Let's face it. This is one of the most controversial sexual topics out there. Once thought to be reserved only for homosexual men, it's slowly becoming more accepted in heterosexual relationships. More and more men are asking "How can I get her to try it?"

SexMYTH: **Too Much Anal Sex Will Cause the Anus to Loosen and You to Have Difficulty Controlling Bowel Movements** Studies are inconclusive on this so it's very important to pay attention to your own body and if you feel any discomfort or have any concerns, stop immediately and see your doctor.

If you happen to be on the receiving end of this question, it can be a very scary idea. You may be thinking:

- "Good girls don't do that."
- "Will it hurt?"
- "Is it safe?"
- "Is there any way that I'm really going to enjoy this?"
- "If I do this once, is he going to want to do it every time?"

The list of questions and concerns goes on and on. . . .

It's not the goal of this book to tell you that you should or should not have anal sex, but we do want to educate you on some backdoor basics so that you can make an informed and educated decision for yourself.

Is It Dangerous?

It can be if not done carefully. The membranes around the anus are very thin and can be torn if you're not careful. Anal sex is not the place for rough or vigorous sex—no exceptions. Nor does the anus produce its own lubricant like the vagina does.

We recommend using a good silicon-based lube or a thick water-based lube for anal sex and plenty of it. Silicon lube does not break down in water the same way a water-based lube will and is great for anal sex, extended play, and certain types of sex toys.

Also, remember that the anus is intended to be an exit point, not an entry point. An important thing to remember is "If you play in the mud, you need to wash up." You cannot, under any circumstances go from anal sex back to vaginal sex. Feces are loaded with bacteria so you run the risk of transferring that bacteria from the anus to the vagina. It is, however, okay to go from vaginal sex to anal sex—just not the other way around.

HE **SAYS . . .**

It's true, guys oftentimes like to play a little harder and rougher, but anal sex is definitely not the place for that. So many men love getting their girl to have anal sex because it's still to some degree a forbidden fantasy, but if you indulge your man, just make sure he goes slow and gentle . . . and indulge sparingly.

And *always* wear a condom, no exceptions. Just like other types of sexual activity, STI's and STD's can be transferred to your partner through anal sex.

Will It Hurt?

If rushed or done too aggressively, anal sex can definitely hurt. It's critical to take your time, go very slowly, and use plenty of lube. In this case, saliva is definitely not enough! How much is too much? That depends on the individual. The important thing is that you pay attention to your body and if there is any discomfort, stop immediately. Warning: *Never* use a numbing lube for anal play, because you might not notice discomfort or pain before the damage is done.

How Can We Make Anal Sex More Enjoyable?

Talk about it. Tell your partner why you want to try anal. Find out why he's interested. He may not even know or it may be one of his biggest fantasies. It's important to know where he's coming from. Just as important: Share your concerns, fears, and desires and talk about how to deal with any concerns that either one of you have before you agree to try anal sex. You should also:

1. **Take it very slowly.** The sphincter muscles around the anus can be very tight, so it's important to relax and spend some extra time massaging the area and giving your muscles time to relax. Try some slow, gentle finger play first and maybe even use a small dildo / vibrator if you're comfortable with sex toys.

2. **Use lots of lube.** We've said it before, but it's worth repeating. If you're going to try anal sex, you need to use lube. Silicon is best but a really thick water-based lube will work, too.

3. **Relax.** If you're relaxed, your anus will relax and insertion will be much easier. If you're tense and resist, it will likely be more painful. If you're a mom, remember your breathing

from childbirth and just relax. This is nothing compared to having a baby!

4. **Communicate.** Tell your partner if it hurts or if he needs to go more slowly. And if it feels good, let him know that too.

5. **Talk about it again.** It's so important to talk about new experiences after the fact. Tell him how you felt, what worked, and what didn't. Find out the same from him. This experience should bring you closer together, whether or not you decide to do it again.

50. *Keep It Clean*

As most things that go without saying, it's probably worth mentioning: Make sure anything you put in your body is clean. No matter what it is, you need to know where it came from, who handled it, how safe it is, and so on. Be extra careful when using homemade sex toys. If you don't know what kind of bacteria is on that cucumber, or how smooth that metallic or glass household item truly is, play it safe. Don't risk it. Here are a few tips for the proper care and handling of your sex toys:

Keep Your Toys to Yourself

We're taught early on to share our toys, but that doesn't always apply to sex toys. Sure various toys can be great fun and can add some spice to your love making with your sex partner(s), but that's where it stops. Don't lend or otherwise share your sex toys.

This is mostly an issue of hygiene and safety. As long as you control your toys, you know where they've been and whether or not they're still safe to use.

Don't Borrow Other People's Toys

For the same basic reasons, don't borrow your friend's cool new sex toys. You don't know where they've been! Actually, you probably have a pretty good idea of *exactly* where they've been. So, hold on to that thought and get your own toy. Seriously, it's worth it.

Wash Your Toys

Be aware of exactly what you're doing with your toy, and clean it after every use. This can be important even during the same play session. If you're exploring one area and have an urge to introduce your Rabbit to another area, take the time to give him a quick bath with a good toy cleaner that is designed specifically for your toy. You'll be glad you did because there's nothing sexy about a yeast infection or worse. Read the label on your particular toys for cleaning directions. Some can be cleaned with just soap and water, some others require a disinfecting cleaner, etc.

51. *Dirty Talk Rocks*

So, your man wants you to talk dirty to him? If you're feeling shy about this, get over it. Men love it when you talk dirty to them. Some men like to have sexual adventures described to them in great detail, others simply like it when you use dirty talk or curse words during sex. Here's how to talk dirty to your man in three easy steps.

1. **Talk about It.** Yes, before you actually try this in action, sit down and talk about what he would like to hear. Depending on how adventurous or conservative he is, you may be

surprised at what he actually finds arousing. Talking about it beforehand can keep you from feeling uncomfortable or embarrassed later. . . .

2. **Relax and Have Fun**. Just be yourself and say what comes naturally. You're probably already thinking it anyway. We all have a bad girl that's just waiting to get out. Now's her chance! A good way to break the ice and get started is to simply tell him what you like during sex and to tell him how good it feels when he does *X*. Men love compliments and this is the perfect time and place to give them.

3. **Experiment with Different Words and Tones.** Now that you're comfortable expressing yourself, start to play with words. You can start by telling him what you like and gradually progress to dirty words and more intense moans. You can even make it a game to see how many different words you can find for various body parts. For example: Breasts can also be called boobs, boobies, titties, jugs, knockers, hooters . . . you get the idea. Search for the words and the tone of your voice that get him the hottest. A great site for this is *www.urbandictionary.com*. Have fun!

HE **SAYS** . . .

Sex is supposed to be fun, so stop taking it so seriously. If something doesn't go the way you envisioned, laugh about it rather than feeling embarrassed. Guys don't care what happened. We're just glad you're in the bedroom with us.

52. *Know What Gets You Hot and Bothered*

Not able to pinpoint exactly what gets you—or your partner—excited? Is it bondage? Role-play? A great way to find out what you like—or love—is to read the following sections, and have your partner do the same, then talk about what turns you both on. How can you incorporate some of these new ideas into your routine without feeling uncomfortable? Well, we guarantee that when you find out what your partner likes, you will open yourself up to it too.

So, yes, your journey toward bringing out your inner pervert has begun—congratulations!

What Types of Personas Turn You On?

You might be really into your partner, but do you sometimes wonder what it would be like to be with someone else? Perhaps you long to be with someone you would probably never be with in real life, like a famous celebrity or athlete? Or, maybe you fantasize about being someone else yourself? Role-playing in bed is a great way to start to let down your sexual inhibitions because you can have fun with the fantasy and play around with power roles. For example, one of you can act as the boss or pilot while the other acts as the assistant or flight attendant or you can have your partner play a persona that turns you on, such as a soldier, firefighter, or even the FedEx guy. Need some ideas? Choose some personas on the following list that turn you on:

- Nurses, doctors, medical professionals.
- Interns/assistant/secretary.
- Cowboys, cowgirls, farmers.
- Truck drivers.

- Religious figures (rabbis, priests, nuns).
- Prostitutes, pimps, sex workers, Johns, sluts.
- Fantasy creatures (mermaids, werewolves, vampires, etc.).

No matter what personas turn you on, don't be embarrassed to talk about them with your partner.

What Clothes Turn You On?

When you go to the store, what fabrics do you generally gravitate to? Or, when you're in a sex shop, what clothing items do you secretly admire? Some of us are turned on by the smell of leather while others love the feel of latex. Does your partner always do a double take when he sees you in his T-shirt? Does he get all hot and bothered when he sees your wearing a certain pair of high heels? Next time you're in the bedroom, take the opportunity to get dressed up. It doesn't have to be as intricate as a full dominatrix outfit complete with laced-up, thigh-high, leather boots (unless that turns you on), but find an outfit that appeals to your lover's tastes . . . or ask him to buy one for you!

Need some ideas? Try the following:

- Rubber, latex.
- Legwear (fishnets, pantyhose, tights).
- High heels.
- Uniforms (UPS, military, servant, schoolgirl).
- Clothing style (Gothic, preppy, etc.).
- Corsets.

Talk to your partner and see if any of these get him going—and vice versa. If so, talk about giving it a try.

What Locations Get You Off?

They always say: "Location, location, location." And, it's true. One of the secrets to keeping your sex life fun is not always having sex in the same place. Consider moving around the house as tables, countertops, the couch, and other household surfaces can work great for sex. You should also consider exploring the outdoors, perhaps making love in the secluded woods behind your house or in the ocean when no one is looking. Go on, be adventurous! Need some ideas? Try the following:

- Bathroom, hot tub.
- Museums, libraries, etc.
- Farms and stables.
- Truck stops.

Feel free to use your imagination and pick a place that works for you!

We Like to Watch

One way to discover your partner's tastes—and for him to discover yours—is to watch porn together. There are some female-friendly adult film directors making movies today and by watching an adult film together, you'll learn what scenes your partner finds most arousing and might find some new moves to add to your own sex life. Some scenes you may find evocative and want to try include:

- Vanilla romance (dinner by candlelight, movie dates, cuddling).
- Having sex in a public place.

- Having rough sex (hair pulling, biting, etc.).
- Playing in combination with other couples.
- Being spanked because you have been a naughty girl.

You might also want to consider making a sex tape or taking sexy photos of your own so you can watch them later and use them as masturbation material. Some other fun things you can try are doing a strip tease for your partner, masturbating in front of your partner (remember, men love visual stimulation), and attending a strip club together and picking out dancers for the other. As long as you can both keep jealousy at bay, the two of you can have fun learning more about the other's sexual appetites.

*Sex*MYTH: **Casual Sex Is Always a Bad Idea for Women**

Women can love casual sex just as much as men. Just because women usually want to feel an emotional connection to fully enjoy sex within a relationship, doesn't mean they can't have as much fun in a one-night stand as men can. So, if there's a guy you find attractive and just want him for the night, have fun, but just be sure to use protection. It doesn't make you promiscuous; it means you're taking charge of your sexual needs!

Tantalize Your Senses

As we mentioned, kitchen gadgets can work great as sex objects, but did you know that you could also use the items in your pantry and freezer as well? Consider covering your lover in chocolate or another creamy delight and licking it slowly off of him. Or, bring all his nerves to a fever pitch by using a candle to pour hot wax on his bare skin or trace an ice cube over his body. Want to kick it up a notch? Try either restraining or being restrained by your partner while you play. Through experimentation, you'll find something that really brings out the animal passion in your lover.

Restrain Me

Tying your partner up or being tied up by your partner can be quite exhilarating. It allows the free partner to be in control of the other's pleasure (or pain, if that's your thing) without the other person stopping him. For example, if you're the kind who always pushes your lover's head away during oral sex when you're about to reach orgasm, try asking him to use handcuffs or a piece of silk to tie your hands together so you can't stop him. You might be quite pleased with the result. To add an extra level of excitement, consider also using a blindfold, as you experience pleasure with the anticipation of not knowing what's coming next. There are a few different ways to use restraint play. Try the following and decide what works for you:

- Being tied up, caressed, and loved.
- Being tied up and tickled.
- Being tied up and (sexually) teased.
- Being tied up in a comfortable position.
- Being tied up in discomfort.
- Being tied up and (in a sexual way) exposed.
- Being tied up and whipped, flogged, or spanked.
- Being restrained and left alone.

A Little Pain, Please

Have you ever noticed when you smack or grab your partner's butt particularly hard during sex he gets even more aroused? Or he moans in pleasure when you drag your nails up his back? Then we suggest it might be time to go to your local sex shop together and consider investing in some bedroom toys. If he likes spanking, think about a paddle, whip, or crop. If he enjoys the sensation of your nails, try a Waternberg wheel. Of course, these are just the basics. Need more ideas? Try the following:

- Nipple clamps and clothespins.
- Whips.
- Paddles.
- Riding crops/flogs.
- Gags.

The sky is the limit, but why not start here?

Turning Fantasy into Reality

If there's something you've been fantasizing about for years, talk to your partner about the possibility of making it a reality if you think it would be something he would accept without hurting your relationship (for example, if your fantasy is having sex with his brother, you might want to leave this one in your head). But if your fantasy is a threesome, or having sex in public, or joining the mile-high club, it might be worth mentioning. He might even have some ideas he's been previously too shy to share with you that you'd love to try. By sharing your fantasy you can help to create an environment of trust and openness with your partner, which includes accepting him and his kinks—even if they're a little outside of your box at first.

Now It's Your Turn

Once you figure out what you like, talk to your partner. You may be surprised at what he says does it for him. Your answers may move you into a realm that you have not explored individually or with your partner.

Remember to truly have the best sex of your life, you have to be willing to let go, try new things, and work through some of your old baggage. You may just surprise yourself if you'll just give it a try. Have fun with the results! Take turns picking a fantasy and trying it out together.

Test Your Comfort Zone

Start small with blindfolds and silk scarves; simple sensory deprivation can be a real turn-on. A friend of mine had no idea she liked blindfolds, until her boyfriend spontaneously wrapped her winter scarf around her head and gave her a massage on the couch. Instant addition to their bag of tricks!

You may find that you like a little smack on the bottom during the heat of the moment or having your hands restrained—or maybe you don't. Maybe you'll discover that the scent of chocolate syrup sends you over the edge or that you really do feel sexy in that French maid outfit? How do you know if you don't give it a try? The important thing is that you are willing to try something new and adventurous. If you do, your sex life will never again be boring.

Be "Try-Sexual"

It pays to try new things, even if you think you might not like them. If you find you're not crazy about something, don't do it again. As long as you keep open communication going, pushing your boundaries shouldn't ruin anything. It's all a learning process.

You can also experiment with swatting the bottom during sex, or pinning your partner's hands above his head while you're making love. Take a candle and drip hot wax on your partner—it's easy to monitor this one—the higher up you hold it above someone when it drips, the less it hurts.

Someone once told me that they loved sex because it reminded them of what it was like to be a kid. "Excuse me?" I said, eyebrows raised. "And just what kind of childhood did you have?" He laughed and explained, "With sex you get to be really messy and play make believe and just have fun!" Make sure whatever you do, you really do have a good time. After all, that's part of what sex is for!

53. He Likes Compliments as Much as You Do

You like to receive compliments from your man (or any man) right? Guess what? He likes compliments as much as you do.

It's important to take the time to tell your man how much you want, need, and love him on a regular basis. Try this. For one whole day, don't say anything negative to your man, don't ask him to do anything, and don't try to fix him. Instead, compliment him on the good things that he does, no matter how small or seemingly insignificant.

Want to make this more of a long-term endeavor? Go out and buy a journal or notebook. Even a piece of paper will work. Every night for a set amount of time, think of at least five things that you like about your partner. You don't have to tell him about these things, just start writing them down. This little exercise will help you remember the things that you do like about him. Once you feel comfortable writing them down, then you can start sharing them with him. Still need ideas? Here are ten ways to compliment your man:

1. **Appreciate Him.** If he takes you out for dinner, tell him how good the food is, how much you like his choice of restaurant, how wonderful it is to spend time with him. If he brings you ice cream from the store, thank him even if it's the wrong flavor. Remember, he took the time to think of you and do something special for you.

2. **Compliment His Relationship Skills.** When he does something special like give you an unexpected hug, bring you flowers, open the car door, or kiss you goodbye, make sure to tell him how much you appreciate it and how much it means to you.

3. **Compliment His Physique or Strength.** Compliment his strength, even if all he did was open the pickle jar. If he works out, let him know that you see improvement, no matter how minor. If you don't see physical changes, compliment his dedication and effort to get in shape.

4. **Compliment His Looks.** Find something about his appearance that you really like and point it out to him, just make sure you don't overdo this one. Tell him you really like his blue eyes, or his broad shoulders, or the way a certain shirt looks on him.

5. **Acknowledge His Successes.** No matter how small the success, men like to feel appreciated. Express sincere interest in something that he values whether it is his work or a certain sports activity. Basically, be proud of him. Not only

tell him, but share his successes with others and let him hear you do it.

6. **Compliment His Intellect.** Tell him how impressed you are that he knows so much about X, Y, or Z. Maybe you and your partner are total opposites? If so, he's likely to know more than you about certain things. Notice these things and point them out.

7. **Compliment Him on a Job Well Done.** Did he fold that load of towels? Did he fix the broken door knob? Did he get a promotion at work? Tell him he did a good job, even if he didn't do it the way you would have.

8. **Compliment His Skill in Bed.** A very large part of a man's sexual satisfaction comes from knowing that he is satisfying his partner. Let him know that you like what he's doing with words or moans—just let him know.

9. **Ask Him for Help.** Ask him to help you solve a problem, carry the groceries, or teach you how to do something. Men love to help and they love to solve problems, so why not give him to opportunity to feel good about himself?

10. **Laugh at His Jokes.** While this may seem silly, it shows that you're paying attention and that you find him funny and interesting. Just be careful not to overdo it. You don't want to sound insincere.

HE **SAYS . . .**

Men absolutely want to feel appreciated. We love to hear the positive, the things that went right, not just what needs fixing.

Watch the change in the way he treats you over the next month or so if you keep it up.

54. *Phone Sex Works! Give It a Try*

Did you know that just because you can't be near your partner doesn't mean you can't keep those sexual fires burning? One great way to do so is by engaging in phone sex with him. It's sort of like talking dirty in bed, but there's more buildup as you both have to set the scene. Ask your partner what he is wearing, where he is, and how much he would like you to touch him while you are on the phone. As things get hotter and you two start masturbating while on the phone with each other, you can tell him what you want him to do to you and what you would do to him if he was there. As you get more hot and bothered, don't be afraid to be vocal. Because even if your partner can't see you, he can still hear you, and it's especially hot for him to hear your pleasure over the phone line.

Sexting

When you send sexual text messages, or sexts, to your significant other, you can get him in the mood for later. Text about what you want to do with him later, or what you're doing that's hot at the moment, or send him a photo of something sexy you are wearing or plan to wear later to help get him in the mood. If you two start sexting back and forth, you may both get so worked up you'll have to take an early lunch for a secret rendezvous!

55. *Watch Yourself Do It*

Have fun with mirrors. Having sex in front of a mirror (or two or three) can be very exciting for both you and your partner. You may feel a little insecure at first but that will quickly be replaced by arousal as you watch your hands move together over one another's bodies.

You may be surprised to learn that sex in front of a mirror can be much sexier than videotaping yourselves in the act. Unless you're a pro, what you see on the video can be less than attractive. It's amazing what goes into creating a video where everyone looks good—especially naked!

56. Talk about Your Sex Life

Women crave intimacy. Men crave ecstasy. But do you really know what your partner wants and needs in bed? How does he know what you really want and need in bed? Simple. You talk about it.

We all know that it's important to communicate our wants, needs, and desires to our partner and vice versa; you simply cannot have a truly amazing relationship or sex life without it. But when it comes to talking about sex, it's often easier to talk to our girlfriends than it is to talk to our partners. Sometimes, it seems that every time you try, it turns into a fight or blame game and someone gets his or her feelings hurt. It may seem easier to keep your mouth shut and hope he reads your mind.

So how do you share your wants, needs, and desires—and listen to your partner—and not crash and burn? Here are a few ground rules that will make the conversation go much better.

Timing Is Everything

Understand that there is a right time and a right place for everything. Bringing up intimate issues in front of the family or friends is never appropriate. Choose a private setting when you're alone together with no distractions. That means no children, pets, ringing phones, or television. It's also a very bad idea to bring up the topic of sex while you're having sex or right after you've had sex. Right before bed is also a bad time to bring it up because you're both tired and ready for sleep.

Why not schedule a date to talk about sex? Go to a neutral place, away from the bedroom, where neither of you feel threatened or intimidated. Go to a nice coffee shop or restaurant where you can have a quiet, private conversation.

HE **SAYS . . .**

I can't say this enough, lying is lying, and it's rarely a good thing. Just like you don't want your man to tell you that you look great in that little dress you had trouble fitting into, he doesn't want you to tell him the sex was amazing if you faked it. Yes, coming clean can be a little awkward, but your lover, your partner, deserves at the very least your honesty. You can be honest without hurting someone's feelings, but do your best to be honest.

If your partner is one of those who storms out of the room every time the conversation gets personal, you may need to go away for the weekend to talk it out. Maybe rent a cabin or boathouse for the weekend. This way your partner will have to stay reasonably close—unless he's a really good swimmer. Plus, being on the water or out in nature is very calming so it creates a great atmosphere to relax, unwind, and enjoy some good conversation.

Honesty Is the Best Policy

Listen, if there's any hope for a long-term, mutually satisfying relationship, both you and your partner need to be completely upfront and honest. This may seem like common sense, but you'd be amazed at how many people choose to tell lies and half truths to their partners, especially about sexual performance. Yes, it may be easier to say, "you're doing a great job" and then fake an orgasm, but you're only cheating yourself if you choose this approach.

Stop Blaming

It's very easy to get into the blame game. In fact, many times people in relationships don't even recognize that they are placing blame on their partners. Statements like the ones below may seem innocent enough, but they're not.

- "Why do you always . . . "
- "You always seem to . . . "
- "When you do X, I feel . . . "
- "I feel that you . . . "

The common thread in all of these statements is the word *you*. Anytime you use *you* in a sentence, the focus is redirected on you. Get it? See how even that sentence may have caused feelings of defensiveness simply because the word *you* was used a number of times?

When talking to your partner, especially about sensitive topics, *you* is the equivalent of pointing a finger at them. And anytime your partner feels blamed, whether intentionally or unintentionally, he'll likely respond defensively; it is just part of our survival nature that has been left over from prehistoric times.

Rather than blaming, talk about your feelings or about a specific event that occurred—not about your partner's role in the feeling or event. While your partner may not like to hear that you're not satisfied sexually, he's still more likely to at least listen if you approach the conversation diplomatically.

Ask and Listen

If you really want to understand your partner both inside and outside of the bedroom, ask him questions and listen closely to his responses. If you find his answers upsetting, do your best not to get defensive or argumentative. He has just as much right to his perspective as you do to yours—even if your perspective of the same event is widely different. Instead of judging, just be a good listener. Doing so will make it more likely that he'll open up more and you'll probably find out why he's been having issues being intimate with you without you accusing him of being that way and starting an argument. If there's one thing guys hate, it's feeling like they're being blamed.

HE **SAYS . . .**

Okay. I admit it. Guys like to be right. But, ladies, you like it too! I think we all need to remember that it's not about being right and justifying why we did or didn't do something that our partner did or did not enjoy. That's part of the silly ego game that all of us (guys or girls) still get into way too often. Let's be grown-ups (I know, it's hard sometimes) and focus on doing better next time so we get a better result. Take the ego out back and bury it (at least for a while)!

After you've been an empathetic listener, you can ask him for solutions—guys love to solve problems—that would make him happy. Ask him what you could do in the bedroom to make him more comfortable. He may ask you the same, or you could—depending on his hang up—let him know what he can add to his regimen to make you even more content between the sheets. As you two share openly about your sex life, it might even lead to new ideas or sex right then and there! But, even if it doesn't, you'll be armed with new knowledge that will definitely make a positive difference in your sex life and get it back on track.

57. Condoms Can Be Sexy

You might be wondering if your partner really *needs* to wear a condom. You know they protect both you and your partner, but your partner doesn't like how they feel and you think they interrupt the experience.

Well, instead of avoiding condom use altogether (not good! we'll discuss it below) try incorporating them into your night. Have fun putting the condom on; make it sexy for your man. After all, just because a condom may slightly decrease the sensitivity experienced during sex, that's no reason to not protect you and your partner. You can still have a lot of fun with condoms—especially flavored ones and those with warming lubricant—and have a satisfying sex life while staying safe.

For some men, condoms are also an excellent way to help prevent premature ejaculation. If he tends to go too quickly, wearing a condom might help him last longer—and ensure that you both reach the finish line. Some condoms are even available with desensitizing gel or cream that will help keep your man from ejaculating too quickly.

So, Do I Need a Condom?

Okay, so condoms can be fun. But does your partner really *need* to wear one? The answer is, yes! Condoms can help prevent pregnancy and STDs. There are a few different types of condoms and some are better at protecting you than others. Animal-skin condoms are too porous to prevent STDs, but they're still effective at preventing pregnancy. Traditional latex condoms are even better at preventing pregnancy and offer good protection against STDs as well.

HE **SAYS . . .**

Honestly, if it was a viable choice, most guys would probably forgo using condoms because they prefer the sensations they feel without them. But, for many couples, that just isn't an option because your man probably doesn't want to get you pregnant (at least not right now) and neither of you wants to end up with an STD. So, don't be shy and just march proudly up to the counter and purchase your condoms. Why not be excited that you're going to get laid soon?

But what if you're on birth control? It depends . . . if you aren't on any other medications (such as antibiotics) that can lessen their effectiveness, you're in a trustworthy monogamous relationship, and you take your birth control at the same time every day, maybe not. But, if all three of those factors don't hold water, then, yes, your partner needs to wear a condom. Not only will you likely prevent yourself from catching a disease, you're that much more likely not to get pregnant.

But I'm Embarrassed to Buy Them . . .

Don't be! If you're buying condoms, it means you're having sex. That's a good thing, right? You can buy condoms at any drug store, supermarket, or convenience store and they're incredibly inexpensive. If you'd like more privacy while purchasing your condoms or would like a wider variety of condoms to choose from, there are many online stores that offer flavored, glow in the dark, colored, and other types of condoms that you and your partner can really have a lot of fun with! If you purchase your condoms online, they'll come to you in discreet packaging and no one will know but you! Honestly though, there's nothing wrong with purchasing condoms, it just means that you're being safe and you're getting ready to have a great time.

All in all, it's important to be safe and it's always better to be safe than sorry, right? But remember to have fun with condoms. Incorporate them into your sex play. After all, if you and your partner make condoms sexy, they will be sexy.

58. Get Kinky and Try Spanking

You'll be hard pressed to find a man who has not fantasized about spanking a woman's bare bottom. But whether this is a kinky fetish for him or simply a creative way to spice it up sexually, spanking can be pleasurable both for him and for you.

HE SAYS . . .

Don't be shy ladies. Men are usually totally on board with this fantasy. Just figure out what side of the fence your man is on. Does he want to tie you up and spank you? Or vice versa? Which arouses you more? It's okay to say "both."

Before you let him spank you (or vice versa), you have to find out if your partner is even open to the idea. If your partner has ever hinted that he might enjoy some dominant/submissive fun, then spanking may well be an option. If there haven't been any obvious hints, then you'll have to find a way to bring it up in conversation.

Here's the thing: Most women (not all) truly do fantasize about being dominated in bed—that's why all of those steamy romance novels are so popular. Can you imagine one of those shirt-tearing hunks being all passive and wishy-washy about what he wants? No way! They know what they want and they take it. However, it works both ways and if your man wants you to try spanking him, why not give it a go?

So, once you and your partner have both agreed that you'd like to give spanking a try, here are some tips to make it pleasurable for both of you.

What Should You Spank With?

There are many different tools out there for spanking—belts, paddles, flogs, whips, etc. The list goes on and on. The all-time favorite for most people (especially in the beginning) is the bare hand. Using your hand (or having your partner use his) allows you both to really feel what's going on and can improve the emotional and mental connection between the two of you.

How to Give a Spanking

Sure, giving a spanking sounds easy, but giving a good, sexually arousing spanking requires a little more thought and preparation. Here are a few things you'll want to remember before bringing your hand to his bottom:

1. **Warm Up.** Make sure that your hands are warm, not cold.
2. **Pick a Hand.** It doesn't matter which hand you use, but you should only use one hand at a time.

3. **Spank One Cheek at a Time.** You should only spank one cheek at a time. Your hand will not make good contact on either cheek if you try to spank them both at the same time.

4. **Check Your Position.** You should be comfortable and your partner's bottom should be easily accessible. You don't want to accidentally smack your partner on the back or too low on the thigh. Remember, we're talking about bottom spanking. Doggie position or straddled over your lap or a stool works very well for this.

5. **Cup Your Hand.** Hold your hand firmly in a slightly cupped position. This will make sure that you get the right impact with the bottom. It should make a good smacking noise and sting just a little. You're not trying to hurt your partner, just to make it sting a little.

6. **Spank It.** Aim for the meatiest part of the bottom and give it a good smack and then rub the area gently to ease the sting before doing it again.

Remember, the person doing the spanking is in control. That's what this fetish is all about! You want to communicate with your partner and make sure that everything is going okay, but don't give up your control by asking things like "Did that hurt?" or "Was that hard enough?" A better option is to come up with some signal before the game begins. Maybe something like moaning and squirming is good. If it's too hard, tap three times.

As always, when you're playing any sort of sexual games, make sure to talk about the experience afterward. How did it go? Did you enjoy it? Do you want to do it again? What did you like the most? What did you like the least? How can you make it better next time?

59. *Stop Smoking for Steamier Sex*

This may be a controversial statement because there are many men out there who feel that the image of a woman smoking a cigarette is incredibly sexy! If you want to light one up occasionally for a little role-play action, have fun. But that's not the point here. This is about the negative side effects that long-term, habitual, addictive smoking have on your sex life.

The negative health effects of smoking have been well-documented. Smoking causes lung cancer, heart problems, and disease of the teeth and gums. Fewer studies have been done on the effects of smoking and libido, but what is starting to be reported does not look good.

HE **SAYS . . .**

In most cases, men who do not smoke (and even some who do) are not looking to date a smoker. In fact, studies have shown that smoking greatly limits your choices when looking for a partner since more and more people perceive smoking as an unattractive, unclean habit. This is particularly true in the United States and Canada. Do yourself (and us) a favor and enhance your love life by putting it out.

It's well known that nicotine weakens the heart and constricts blood vessels. So it only seems logical that the decreased blood flow impacts the flow of blood to both the female and male genitalia, negatively affecting the libido. Another common side effect of nicotine addiction is increased stress and nervousness, both of which have been shown to reduce libido in men and women. This doesn't even take into account the obvious self-esteem issues, another libido buster, that many smokers face—yellow teeth and fingers, excessive coughing and phlegm, and the intense odor that is very noticeable to nonsmokers, all contribute to negative self-image in smokers.

As you can see, except for the occasional usage in role-play and fetish scenarios, smoking is definitely *not* sexy. So, if you are a smoker, give it up and watch your sex drive skyrocket! Trust us, it's worth it.

60. *Give Your Partner the Ultimate Sexual Experience*

If you want to give your lover a night he'll never forget—one he'll remember not just for days, but for years, and have to do his absolute best to resist blogging about—keep on reading.

Do you not think that type of ecstasy is possible? Or if it is, do you think you need to be some kind of expert lover to do it? Well, put your doubts to rest, because the following recommendation will intensify your relationship both in and out of the bedroom, and it's easy to do!

That's right. I'm talking about tantric massage.

What Is Tantric Massage?

Tantric massage may sound intimidating, but, in actuality, it's not all that hard to learn. Tantric massage was developed centuries ago in Asia as a ritual that helped to balance out a person's emotional and physical energy. Reportedly this balance led to healing, tranquility, and the kind of sack sessions that would make Casanova jealous. As an additional bonus, tantric massage can also melt away tension and free your partner's mind from the stress of daily life, thus increasing his—and your—chances of achieving a bed-shattering orgasm.

While the actual practice can take a very long time to master (some followers have been perfecting their techniques for decades), here are a few tricks and tips that you can easily use tonight to give your partner a tantric massage that will blow his mind (and other parts of his anatomy).

Set the Mood

Before you can begin your tantric massage journey, you have to set the proper mood. You don't have to sprinkle rose petals over your bed, but a few changes to your normal bedroom atmosphere will work wonders.

HE SAYS . . .

Ladies, I can't say this enough: Keep it simple. Men love trying new things in the bedroom, but anything that requires an instruction manual is a bit much. Also, overcomplicating something basically ensures that we'll put it off and will never get started—and we want to get started. So, remember, a small step is the best way to slowly achieve great results.

Dim the lights, light a few candles, and play music that's tranquil and soothing (try to avoid any music that has a rhythmic beat). If you normally make love on ordinary cotton sheets, try swapping them for a set with a luxurious thread count or, for a more affordable option, use sheets made from jersey material, which feel silky and smooth against bare skin.

Your lover will definitely appreciate the time you took to set the mood!

Grab the Massage Oil

Once you've set up your bedroom to max out your lover's tantric experience, grab some massage oil, and have your partner remove his clothing and lay face-down on the bed (if you don't want oil on your sheets, place a towel between your lover and the bed).

Pour a few drops of oil in the palm of your hands and rub them together in order to properly warm the oil. After all, nothing can break a sensual mood more than a few drops of something ice cold.

Gently Begin the Massage

Remember, tantric massage is very different from a typical back-and-shoulder rub, so avoid focusing on loosening up knotted muscles. Instead, focus on the feeling of your lover's skin as you glide your hands back and forth along his back. Work your way down to your lover's buttocks and legs as you gently rub your hands in an up-and-down stroking motion. Remember to ask your partner if your touch is too soft or too hard!

After massaging your lover's back, have him turn over onto his back. Begin to gently massage his chest and stomach. Pay attention to sensitive areas, such as your partner's nipples, but don't overtly focus on them, as this could lead to lovemaking too quickly.

Massage Down There

When you reach your partner's privates, be sure to softly massage them as well, but again, at this point, be sure to focus more on the act of the tantric massage and not on pursuing an orgasm.

Enjoy!

Afterward

Once you've completed your tantric massage, your partner will be both relaxed and aroused, which is an ideal physical and mental state for achieving the kind of spiritual orgasm that will make your relationship unbreakable.

However, keep in mind that you shouldn't engage in tantric massage with the expectation that intercourse will always follow. Sex should be a pleasurable bonus, not a final destination. Most importantly, have a fun and positive attitude while giving your partner a tantric massage. Devoting yourself to your lover's pleasure is a beautiful experience, so don't take yourself so seriously. After all, if you're too busy focusing on whether or not it will lead to sex or whether you're doing it correctly, you'll cheat yourself out of the opportunity to engage in one of the most pleasurable and spiritual rituals of tantra!

61. There's More Than One Kind of Orgasm

There is much debate about the different types of orgasms that a woman can have. The four most common are:

- The clitoral orgasm.
- The vaginal orgasm.
- The G-spot orgasm.
- The anal orgasm.

These different types of orgasms really just refer to the area of the body being stimulated. However, it is true that different types of stimulation to different body parts can result in different feeling orgasms for most women.

What's the Difference Between a Clitoral and a Vaginal Orgasm?

This is one of the most common questions about the female orgasm. The difference between a clitoral and a vaginal orgasm is based purely on which body part is stimulated to achieve orgasm.

Many women achieve orgasm when only the clitoris is stimulated or with only vaginal penetration, but the most common way for a woman to experience orgasm is with a combination of clitoral stimulation and either oral sex or vaginal penetration.

There are a number of ways to stimulate your clitoris, including:

- Rubbing.
- Sucking.
- Body pressure.
- Using a vibrator.

*Sex*MYTH: **Vaginal Orgasms Feel Better Than Clitorial Orgasms** It's also been said that vaginal orgasms are more mature than clitoral orgasms. We think all orgasms feel amazing and that it's a personal preference on which feels better. If you find yourself screaming louder when your G-spot is being stimulated than when your partner is paying attention to your clitoris or vice versa, then have that kind of sex!

Your clitoris can also be stimulated during sexual intercourse, most often when you are on top where you can rub your clitoris against your man's pubic bone. You or your partner can also stimulate your clitoris with your fingers or with a vibrator during intercourse. And while many women touch the glans (that little bump) of the clitoris to become aroused, for some that level of direct contact can be too intense.

What Is a G-spot Orgasm?

Most vaginal orgasms are achieved with G-spot stimulation. The G-spot is a very sensitive zone about two or three inches inside the vagina on the front wall, closest to the clitoris or pubic bone. It feels ridged or bumpy—some compare it to the size and shape of a walnut. Rubbing or massaging this area during sex will result in a G-spot orgasm.

Orgasms and the type of stimulation that you prefer are simply a matter of personal preference; there is no one correct way to have an orgasm. No matter how you think of it, orgasms are achieved by stimulating various parts of the body that you find arousing.

While it's easy to get fixated and frustrated if you are unable to have a vaginal orgasm, or because you've never experienced a G-spot orgasm, in reality, different women are aroused in different ways. While it's important to understand all the different parts and myriad techniques used to reach your peak, the best advice is to drop the labels and to do what feels good at the moment.

HE SAYS . . .

Studies show that the percentage of women who have never had an orgasm is staggering. Trust me when I tell you that most guys don't really care *at all* what type of orgasm you have, as long as you just have one! We love getting off, but we're at our best when you're having fun too!

What Is an Anal Orgasm?

As you may have already suspected, an anal orgasm is different from a clitoral or vaginal orgasm. When the anus is being stimulated—either externally or internally—you may experience contraction in the sphincter or surrounding muscle tissues that give the intense feeling of orgasm. And, depending on the position, your partner might even be able to stimulate your G-spot while inside your anus, which can also result in a powerful orgasm.

62. Use Steamy (Instant) Messages to Seduce Your Man

Gone are the days when lovers used pen and ink to write each other careful letters declaring their affections for one another. Modern lovers no longer have the patience to wait for a message to be delivered by postal mail, nor should they have to.

HE **SAYS . . .**

Seeing a woman take some of the initiative is a huge turn-on! It's so great to see you engaged in sex too, instead of just always waiting for us to pursue you. I love to see enthusiasm and initiative on a lady's side.

The Internet, texting, and instant messaging have, in some ways, made our lives more impersonal, but with some creativity you can also use these modes of communication to send some really steamy messages!

Here are some sexy ways to use modern technology to seduce your man:

- **Sexy Text Messages:** If you have a sudden sensual or romantic thought while at work, send him a short text message sharing exactly what you were thinking.
- **Erotic Instant Messages:** Instant messaging is a great way to share some of your more detailed fantasies. It's amazing

how women tend to take on a completely different, and often more flirty and seductive, persona over IM than they do in person.

- **Romantic E-mails:** A spontaneous romantic e-mail is a simple, effective way to show your significant other that you are thinking of him no matter where you are. And with the ability to attach images, video, and music, e-mail has taken the old-fashioned love letter into a whole new realm.

63. Turn the Temperature Up—or Down—for Hot Sex

One thing you've probably learned already is that men and women get cold and hot at different temperatures. What might seem comfortable to a man might feel downright chilly to you and what feels comfortable for you might make a man feel like he's burning up. But what you probably don't know is that temperature can have a big impact on both you and your partner's levels of sexual arousal.

Cozy up to Each Other

Even with people who prefer it warm, turning down the temperature can heat up the sex. If you're the type to get cold easily, we wouldn't recommend having sex outdoors in the winter, but you can take advantage of cool days and nights by cuddling up with your partner and sharing your body heat . . . and more. The next time you're spending the night in the chilly months, invite your partner to share the couch with you and cuddle up together underneath a big blanket. It won't be long, especially with a little initiating on your part, before you're doing more than cuddling!

Heat Up Those Coals

If you find it easier to get in the mood when your body is warm, then by all means, turn up the heat or stoke that fire. If your partner gets warm easily, suggest a clothing-free night or dress only in your lingerie and encourage him to wear something you find equally sexy. If he finds that you're more inclined to dress in sexier clothing or lingerie when the temperature is higher, there's a good chance he'll handle being warm with aplomb.

64. Position Yourself for Pleasure: Get Kinky with Girl on Top

This position looks just like it sounds. You're on top, straddling your partner's hips for penetration. This is one of our favorites because you have so much more control over both the depth and angle of penetration—a must-have for good G-spot and clitoral stimulation. Your breasts and clitoris are also easily accessible and you can go at the speed that feels just right.

To initiate this position, silently put your partner on his back, or, when you two are both naked, ask him to lie down so he's facing you. Then, climb on top of him and slowly slide him inside. Though this position—unless you're facing his knees (learn more about Girl on Top (Reverse) in Entry # 5)—doesn't allow him to penetrate as deeply as other positions do, it does allow you to be in more control of the speed and pressure. And, he's going to certainly love the view of your breasts bouncing in front of him and grabbing your ass as you thrust up and down. It doesn't get much better than that!

65. *Letting Him Look but Not Touch Is a Total Turn-On*

You know by now that men are very visual creatures. But being able to look but not touch really heightens their arousal. And you can use this knowledge even before you get into bed. If you are kissing him, don't allow him to kiss you back. Kiss his lips and run your tongue around them but tell him he can't do the same. You'll soon notice he'll be aching to kiss you back. Try adopting a classic strip club move and give him a lap dance or a sexy strip tease without permitting him to make a move on you. It won't be long until he can't hold his composure any longer and the two of you end up in bed, or at the very least, fondling each other and kissing passionately. There's a reason that strip clubs and burlesque shows are so popular, and it's not just because men like seeing naked women. They love the art of the tease—so remember that the next time you have a chance to take it slow and you'll be pleased with the intensity of his desire.

66. *Contraception Is a Great Wingman*

When you have sex with someone for the first time, there usually isn't a lot of talking. Instead, the two of you will use body language and eye contact to move from the couch to the bedroom and from fully clothed to undressed. And when it comes to the part where contraception is important, all one of you has to do is pull out a condom and the other can simply give a nod.

Safe sex is sex that you don't have to worry about, leaving your mind open to focus solely on experiencing the pleasure to come. So, do yourself a favor and keep the following tips in mind to help ensure that the mind-blowing sex you have with your new flame is safe as well as red-hot.

Don't Rely on Your Partner

Having safe sex is your responsibility. Don't expect your lover to bring condoms or to ask if you are on the pill. Instead, protect yourself from getting pregnant or catching an STD and come prepared. It'll save you from having unsafe sex or having no sex at all. And, if both of you end up bringing contraception, you can always save the spare for another romp.

HE **SAYS** . . .

Ladies, it's your responsibility to have protection (condoms) with you just as much as it is the man's. Frankly the downside for not having one is way worse for you, after all, your partner is not the one who's going to get pregnant! So, leave the "but the man should do that" excuses at the door and take control of your life. Men and women are finally seen as equals. Take full and total responsibility for your choices. You will be surprised how much better your life actually is.

Make a Joint Decision

We have some bad news. Even though we're way into the new millennium, guys are still in the dark ages when it comes to putting condoms on during sex. Oftentimes, men (no matter how much they care about you or want to protect themselves) will still put the responsibility on you to pause sex so they can slip one on instead of bothering to put one on themselves. It goes back to that issue of guys not really wanting to wear condoms even though they know they are in their best interest.

HE **SAYS . . .**

Having sex without a condom feels great, but it is certainly anything other than safe. Unfortunately, the number of teens having sex using the pulling out or withdrawal method is incredible. Having your partner pull out in time is *not* safe sex because there is no point that is truly in time. You can get STDs, STIs, and you can still get pregnant even if your man pulls out before he shoots off! Make sure your man wears a condom, every single time!

If you find yourself in this situation, you know that you are every bit as impassioned as your partner, and should not be the only one who decides whether or not contraception will be used. After all, how are you supposed to let go and enjoy yourself if all the responsibility falls to you. Instead, talk to your partner about safe sex during a nonsexual, calm moment together before it's necessary for you to be the responsible one in the relationship. Knowing that issue is off the table will make things go smoother when the moment does happen and you will be able to stop worrying about stopping and start focusing on enjoying the ride. But, what if your man still isn't into slipping on a condom before you get going? Well, if he is not willing to share the responsibility, maybe he shouldn't be the one sharing your bed.

Sperm, Semen, and Safe Sex: What You Need to Know

These terms are thrown around as if they're common knowledge, but the fact is that very few people actually know how they differ, which can be dangerous for your health, and lead to confusion in the bedroom—not what you want when you're looking to get off. So, learn these terms and take the pressure out of sex by knowing what you're dealing with in the bedroom:

- **Pre-cum:** The clear, thinnish, and somewhat sticky liquid that comes out of the head of the penis in small amounts during penile stimulation before he actually ejaculates. Pre-cum can and often does contain live sperm, although in significantly smaller amounts than actual semen.
- **Semen:** The whitish, thicker fluid that comes out of the head of the penis during ejaculation. Semen contains millions of sperm.
- **Sperm:** Reproductive cells carried within semen and pre-cum that join with a woman's egg to conceive a child.

Which of These Can Get You Pregnant?

In short—all of them!

Pre-cum and semen both contain sperm. Having unprotected sex without a condom, even before your man ejaculates, can get you pregnant. Many women believe that allowing a man to have intercourse with her without a condom is a sound contraceptive, as long as the guy pulls his penis out of her vagina before he ejaculates, and ejaculates away from her vagina. While this method is safer than allowing your partner to actually ejaculate inside you, it is not a way to protect against pregnancy. Instead, it is better to treat a penis like a loaded gun. Understand that sperm can travel out of the penis pretty much at any time and allowing a condomless penis to get anywhere near the vicinity of your vagina puts you at a definite risk of getting pregnant.

So, don't chance it! Even allowing your partner to rub his penis on the outside of your vagina without a condom can transmit sperm and there's a reason that they are called little swimmers. They travel! For the safest type of sex, always use a condom and put it on early. You can also discuss with your doctor other methods of birth control that can be used in conjunction with a condom for added protection, or in lieu of a condom if you are with an STD-free partner and in a completely faithful, monogamous relationship.

Which of These Can Transmit a Sexually Transmitted Disease?

In short—all of them!

Again, treat a condomless penis like a loaded gun, even more so if you're unsure if your partner has a sexually transmitted disease. To clarify, unless you have a piece of paper in your hand that says your partner has tested negative for STDs and you're 110 percent positive your partner has not had any type of sexual contact with anyone else since the test was taken, you're unsure of whether your partner has an STD. Protect yourself. Both precum and semen can carry the HIV-AIDS virus, as well as other STDs. While both fluids can cause pregnancy, it is important to be even more vigilant if you're concerned about STDs because you also have to worry about these fluids possibly coming into contact with your mouth or any open sores or cuts on your body.

For example, if you nicked yourself shaving and your partner rubs his penis up your leg without a condom, you can possibly contract an STD that way. It's rare, yes. But it is possible. Be safe and get tested, suggest that your partner get STD-tested, stay in a monogamous, faithful relationship whenever possible, and use condoms during anal sex, oral sex, and vaginal intercourse any time you're unsure. Always treat your partner's penis as though it can get you pregnant or give you an STD because, in truth, it can! That doesn't mean you can't enjoy sex—and, in fact, you'll enjoy sex even more if you feel comfortable and confident with your partner. Just be safe and be smart about it!

67. Sex Toys Can Strengthen Your Orgasm

Can sex toys really help you achieve stronger orgasms? Absolutely!

Adding sex toys to your sexual play can not only increase the strength of your orgasms, but can help you experience different types of orgasms that you may not be able to experience through traditional masturbation, intercourse, or oral sex. And for those women who tend to take a really long time to reach orgasm through traditional methods, toys just may be the solution.

*Sex*MYTH: **Masturbation Produces the Best Orgasms** This one depends on a number of factors. How skilled are you at pleasuring yourself? How in tune are you sexually with your partner? How adept is your partner at helping you to reach orgasm? If you don't have much experience masturbating and your partner is a pro at oral sex, we have a feeling the orgasm is going to be better with him. The answer to this all depends on your situation.

Vaginal Orgasm with a Vibrator

If you can easily orgasm from direct clitoral stimulation, but never seem to have an orgasm during intercourse, using a vibrator can help. Rabbit vibrators work great for this because they have a shaft for vaginal stimulation and a clitoral stimulator that work together to bring you to orgasm.

These vibrators merge the familiar feeling of teasing your clitoris and add the thrusting effect inside your vagina. The end result is often amazing. Many women claim to have their most powerful and intense orgasms with their Rabbits! However other women claim that the stimulation from this type of vibrator is just too intense. You'll have to try one out for yourself to determine what works best for you personally.

*Sex*MYTH: **A Man Should Be Able to Last More Than Twenty Minutes During Sex** This goes back to the old vaginal-sex-is-the-only-sex idea. Today, sex is about so much more than penetration. Some men last thirty seconds and others can go all night. Neither of these are ideal, so it's important to work with your partner to find what works for both of you. Also, don't forget about oral sex, clitoral stimulation, and masturbation; there are many, many different ways to enjoy yourselves sexually. Try to enjoy them all and put the stopwatch away.

G-spot Vibrators

Still trying to figure out how to have a G-spot orgasm? It can often seem like an impossible task, but G-spot vibrators are here to save the day! As their name suggests, these vibrators are designed to stimulate the G-spot. They have a curved end that easily hits that small spot and makes what was once nearly impossible, an absolute breeze. By moving the vibrator around and changing the pressure, you will find what sort of stimulation works best for you. Plus, a little practice with this toy will certainly help when your partner is in the bedroom because you'll know exactly where your own G-spot is and how to guide your man to it.

Multiple Orgasms with a Vibrator

Most women can experience more than one orgasm during a single sex session. This task, however, can be exhausting for your partner. It is much easier to have multiple orgasms with a vibrator since it never gets tired and, with enough batteries on hand, can give you as many orgasms as you can stand.

With multiple orgasms practice makes perfect. The trick is to keep going after you've had your first orgasm. It may also require a different type of stimulation. For example if you just reached orgasm by stimulating your clitoris, it may be too sensitive for more action right away, so you may want to switch over to your favorite G-spot vibrator or turn the ears off on your Rabbit.

68. *Keep the Spark Alive*

Many people find themselves in relationships where the spark has all but died out. As unfortunate as it is, if you're not getting it on, you're not alone. Does that mean you have to live with it? Of course not! Here are some great ways to understand what is happening in your relationship and what you can do to fix it so you can turn the heat back up.

HE **SAYS . . .**

Guys love sex, but we don't have to have it every day to be satisfied. For most men, it's not about quantity, it's about quality—how great and satisfying the sex is when we do have it. That said, if you're feeling that you're not having sex often enough, your guy is probably more than willing to solve that problem.

What's Your Magic Number?

Different couples have sex at different frequencies. Some have sex once a week and they're completely satisfied. Other couples have sex twice a week and they're not satisfied; they feel like they should be having sex three or four times a week or even every day. Whatever frequency of sex that makes you and your partner most comfortable and satisfied is your magic number. Don't feel that you need to keep up with the Joneses and have more sex than anyone you know. Have sex as often or as little as it takes to keep both you and your partner happy and satisfied!

HE **SAYS . . .**

Men have high sex drives. It's true! And, if their wives or girl-friends put the brakes on regular sex, it's easy for men to take care of their needs in other ways, sometimes to the detriment of their relationships. For example, a guy might get used to masturbating with porn at the same time every evening and, before you know it, he does not want to have sex with his wife since his sex drive is being, well, addressed to some degree. This isn't malicious, just a bad habit that needs to be corrected before it gets out of hand and harms the relationship.

Rev Up Your Sex Drive

The reality is that most men do have a biologically higher sex drive than most women. Unfortunately, this can lead to dissatis-faction on the man's part. The good news is that today's women want sex more and more than in the past. It was only a few months ago that I was at a party where five women out of the five couples in attendance were unhappy with the amount of sex they were getting. If this sounds like you, talk to your partner about it. After all, he won't know you want it if you don't let him know.

HE **SAYS . . .**

Okay, ladies, I'm just going to lay it out for you. I mean no disrespect to your men, but in many ways, a man is like a puppy. He wants really badly to please you and if you tell him good boy when he did it wrong (e.g., faking an orgasm), he'll keep doing it wrong to please you over and over again. But if you're honest and train him right, he'll do his very best to keep you satisfied.

Stay Connected

Clearly there are some serious problems with couples knowing how to stay connected emotionally and sexually. Women tend to be more aware of their emotional needs and men tend to be more aware of their sexual needs, but this does not mean that men and women are set up for failure. Both parties have to be willing to respect and have empathy for each other's needs. To do this, you have to get out of the blame game and stop seeing your partner as the bad guy.

Honestly, sometimes you really do have to be willing to stretch out of your comfort zone sexually in order to have the kind of connection you want with your partner. Don't do something that you find painful or embarrassing, but push your boundaries and try something new if it's what your man wants. He should do the same thing for you, too. And, if either you or your partner finds that sex is not fun, then you *must* take personal responsibility for making sure that changes. To do this, you must respect your partner enough to speak your truth and not fake orgasms. The biggest drain on sexual communication and satisfaction is faking it. How in the world is your lover ever going to know what you want if you pretend you like something you don't?

Learn to get great sex by being open with your truths. You want your man to share with you emotionally? Then don't be afraid to be open about what pleases you sexually and what doesn't. After all, oftentimes talking about sex leads to having sex. And being open about and fixing any issues that you're having in the bedroom will ensure that your spark never gets close to going out.

69. Role-Play It Up

You hear these comments all the time:

- "She's playing games with him."
- "He's playing games with her."
- "They're playing games with each other."

And the way it's said makes it all sound so *wrong*. . . .

But if I enjoy a game of tennis with my partner, that seems to be perfectly acceptable. So what's the difference? Nothing, really. You just need to make sure that you play by the rules, no matter what type of game you're playing. Mind games don't always have to be bad. But they can go awry when the people playing the games are playing by a different set of rules, or worse yet, no rules at all.

Playing mind games in love and sex can be everything from exhilarating to heart crushing and can involve anything from psychological bantering to role-playing. The perception that playing mind games is bad comes from the fact that far too many people use little-known seduction tactics to take advantage of other people.

However, when everyone involved knows that they're playing, it can be an incredibly fun ride, a chance to let your hair down and try something new or be someone new for a little while.

One word of caution for couples who like to play games: Make sure that you're always on the same page and are being completely open and honest with one another. If a game goes too far, make sure your partner knows how you feel. If you want it to go farther, let him know that, too.

HE **SAYS . . .**

During role-play, ask yourself, "Am I playing a fun, sexy, arousing game with my man, or am I playing a game against him?" Men want to play, but we want to make sure we're playing together. If you make sure that happens, the experience can be amazing, fun, and very stimulating for your sex life. After all, even if you're flirting with someone else at a bar, your man may be okay with it because he knows he's having really hot sex tonight—with you! The key here is that you need to have a completely open and honest relationship and communicate about your behavior and actions.

Role-Play for Beginners

Want to try role-play, but aren't sure where to begin? Well, here are some brainstorming ideas for coming up with your role-play fantasy:

- Who do you want to be? Define your character in detail. Your character can be anything from a bunny or squirrel to a comic book character. There really are no limits here.
- What's the scenario? Define the scene. Some popular role-play scenes are being arrested by a big strong police

officer, interactions between a boss and secretary, or even rape scenes. Talk about it with your partner and choose something that turns you both on.

- Do you need props or costumes? What will you wear? Will you need handcuffs or a blindfold? Get everything ready in advance so that when the time comes, you can relax and play the game.

- What's your motivation? Experimentation? Submission? Domination? Exhibitionism? Understand why you want to play this game and what will need to happen for it to be a success.

- What are the ground rules? Clearly define what's okay and what's not. That way no one gets hurt (at least any more than they want to) either emotionally or physically.

Role-play can be anything from having an affair with each other to dressing up in a costume and pretending to be a French maid or naughty schoolgirl. The important thing is that you talk about the rules and set boundaries before you begin. And once you get into character, do your best to stay in character until the scene is played out. But above all else, be creative. Don't take yourself too seriously. And have fun!

70. *Experience the Beach in the Buff*

Who doesn't love the beach? The salty surf. The gritty sand. The untamed waves. There's nothing like nature to bring your passionate side to the forefront. So, take the next step and experience nature in the nude. There's absolutely nothing wrong with the human body. It a beautiful creation that should be celebrated and if you're not comfortable in your own skin—just your skin and nothing else—then you will always hold back out of fear of being judged for not living up to someone else's expectations.

Whether or not you decide to join the nudists on the beach, find a way to get comfortable in your own skin. You are truly a beautiful person, so love your body the way your partner does—inside and out!

HE **SAYS . . .**

It sounds corny, but before you can really love someone you must first truly love yourself. Men love women who know who they are and accept themselves, jiggly bits, wide hips, and all. Accept and love yourself first and many of the problems in your life will vanish, as if by magic.

71. *Go Back to Basics*

Vaginal intercourse may not be the only way to have sex, but it is critical to a mutually satisfying sexual relationship. Done the wrong way it can be boring at best and painful at worst. Done the right way, it can be incredibly orgasmic!

Here are some tips to help make vaginal intercourse better for both you and your partner.

Focus on Foreplay

Plenty of warm-up time is crucial, especially for women, and foreplay can include anything from flirting and teasing to oral sex and fingering. The important thing is to do some sort of foreplay long enough for you to become thoroughly wet and aroused. If you have vaginal sex before you are ready, it can be very painful and even tear the vaginal walls. Most women will normally produce enough lubrication for the penis to easily enter their vagina when they're aroused, but this is not always the case. If lubrication is a problem for you, know that there can be many reasons for the lack of vaginal fluid—everything from medical to psychological reasons, to just being too tired. If this is a recurring problem or you're concerned, please see your doctor. For those occasional times when you feel a little dry in the beginning of vaginal sex or during longer sex play, feel free and encouraged to use a good, water-based lube.

Consider Lube

We discussed lube in more detail in Entry # 46, but it's important enough to mention here, too. We want to remind you that water is not a lubricant and neither is saliva (unless you're going down on your man, in which case, we'll make an exception to the rule).

HE **SAYS . . .**

Guys love to look forward to something, particularly something exciting like a night of hot sex. To get your partner in the right frame of mind in time, tease him about it early in the day. He's going to be thinking about sex anyway, why not get him fantasizing about doing things with (and to) you?

Even if lubrication has never been an issue for you, the fact is that sexual lubricants last much longer than what your body produces and if they start to dry out, a few drops of water (even saliva) will reactivate them.

Here are a few really good reasons to get comfortable with lube:

- Lube is a great idea if you're in the mood for a quickie—just because it's spur of the moment doesn't mean that it has to be uncomfortable.
- Lube can prevent tears in the vagina during extended or rough sex.
- Lube makes playing with toys way more fun—this is one situation where water and saliva just won't work.
- Lube is absolutely necessary for anal sex because your anus does not produce its own lubrication.
- Enhancing lubes can sensitize or desensitize as necessary and even add a pleasant scent or flavor to your sexual play.

Get into Position

There are literally hundreds of sexual positions that you and your partner can experiment with. You'll find plenty scattered throughout this book, but it's important to try several until you and you partner find the ones that match your sexual style. Ask yourself, does that position:

- Match your stamina?
- Provide an appropriate level of physical difficulty?
- Improve your chance of orgasm?
- Extend your partner's ability to refrain from orgasm?

Yes, there are positions that can help in all of these areas. Start with the basics and gradually work up to more creative positions. Above all, experiment and have fun.

Keep Up the Rhythm and Pressure

Another important thing to experiment with during vaginal sex is rhythm and pressure. Different women (and men) like different feelings. Some like it hard and fast and others like it slow and rhythmic. And it can change from one sex session to the next. This is why communication is *so* important between you and your partner. It's okay to say things like: "Slow down" (especially if you feel him losing control and you're not ready), "speed up," "harder," "stay there," and "don't stop."

Verbal feedback is very important to make sure that your partner is moving in a way that brings you pleasure. He really does want to make you happy, but you have to speak up. If you don't, you'll only be hurting yourself!

Play with Toys

Another great way to improve vaginal intercourse is the addition of your favorite sex toy. It could be anything from a simple clitoral vibrator or cock ring, to something more extreme like vibrating anal beads or a 10-inch steel dildo.

HE **SAYS** . . .

Some men may be threatened by your sex toys, but those men don't realize how much fun they're missing out on. Sex toys can be great fun to use as a couple—don't just use them to masturbate in the dark when nobody's looking!

Remember what it was like when you were a child and you got a new toy? It was fun, right? You could not wait to play with it. That's how you should approach sex toys. Don't be embarrassed by them. Playing with toys does not mean that your partner is not able to please you and you're no more likely to get addicted to your vibrator than you are to your hair dryer. Toys are just another way to have fun and spice up your sex life. They don't provide the emotional connection that's so crucial in a relationship. Women who say "I don't need a man, I have a vibrator" are only kidding themselves and the people they're saying it to. So relax and enjoy yourself.

72. Fulfill Your Freaky Fantasies

Sure sex feels good on its own, but have you ever thought about taking it up a notch and pushing your boundaries with BDSM—Bondage & Discipline / Domination & Submission / Sadism & Masochism? Do you have any freaky fantasies that might be ready to leave your head? If so, prepare yourself for a challenge. Get off your butt and onto your hands and knees and grab a candle to light the way—just don't forget to let some of the hot wax drip on your sensitive flesh.

As you read through this section, pay attention to your feelings. Which concepts intrigue you the most?

Bondage

When most people think of bondage, the first thing that comes to mind is tying someone to the bedposts or putting on a blindfold. But bondage is truly an art form and many people even make a lifestyle of it, but in its simplest forms it's nothing more than incorporating restraint into lovemaking, then giving yourself over to the pleasure and entrusting yourself to your partner. Bondage play can be as simple as your partner holding your hands together during sex or using blindfolds and handcuffs, and can range all the way to the more complicated forms of Shibari, the art of Japanese Bondage. There are no rules other than the ones you and your partner set before you start.

Being tied up or otherwise restrained can feel scary, relaxing, embarrassing, arousing, or intense. Because of the array of emotions that will definitely come with this type of sexual play, communication with your partner is critical. This is a game of trust. (Read that again.) This is a game of trust. Please talk with your partner about your personal limits and boundaries with this type of role-play. While bondage may sometimes look and feel like forced sex, it's not really forced sex; rather it's a game with rules that both you and your partner need to agree on and adhere to.

HE SAYS . . .

Though not all men are into being tied up and whipped—or enjoy doing those things to their partner—those of us who do love it find it hot for a variety of reasons. For one, it's quite sexy for our partner to be in control and do the initiating. Call us lazy, but sometimes it's a real treat to lie back and be pleasured without the pressure of having to reciprocate. We love to know what our ladies would do to us if they were given complete control. And when we are the ones in charge, it's a rush to watch our partners squirm and moan as we pleasure them all the way to orgasm and beyond all on our own.

Because it is a role-play game, define the rules of the game before you play and make sure to take it slow. And always have a safe word (or gesture if your mouth will be gagged). This is simply a word or gesture that means "Stop, I've had enough."

What Should You Use?

Nylon rope is a good option for bondage because it's cheap or easily obtained at any hardware store. However, beginners often start with silk scarves, neckties or fuzzy handcuffs. Many of the more experienced folks opt for hemp rope, which is available online and in sex shops in a variety of colors. Remember, if it works for you, it's okay! This is your game and you get to make all the rules.

Discipline

Discipline is often used during domination / submission role-play and is basically the use of rules and punishment to control the behavior of someone else—the submissive. A rule can be as simple as not allowing someone to say "thank you" for the evening, and if they transgress, punishment ensues.

What is the first thing that comes to mind when you think of the word *punishment*?

Spanking, perhaps? Certainly, but punishment needn't be physical. BDSM can be extremely creative, not to mention mental.

A typical scenario might be that of King or Queen and a servant where the servant has certain rules to follow. If any of the rules are broken he must be punished. Or it could be the scenario of a Cop and a hooker, where she has to provide sexual favors as discipline to repay her crimes. It could even be that the submissive is not allowed any sexual gratification until the master allows it. The list goes on and on and is only limited by your imagination both for the scenario and the punishments. It can be as easy or hard as you want it to be.

Domination

Domination is exercising control over others. The person who exercises that control is commonly called the Dom, Master, Mistress,

Boss, or Top. A Dom is in charge, gives orders, calls the shots, and administers the punishments. But, whether you or your partner are playing this role, the Dom has to have the right balance of kindness and meanness, kind of like that tough love you hear about when it comes to parenting teenagers. An example of a good Dom move would be giving the Sub a good smack on the rear, and then tenderly kissing the sting away.

Does it sound like the Dom can do whatever the hell she wants? Think again. Ultimately, the play session is limited to what the Submissive is willing to do. Communication is key, so discussing ahead of time what is on the sexual menu and what is off limits is critical. Important note: Being a Dom is not an excuse to be a jerk.

Submission

Submission is the desire to be dominated and have control exercised over you. Also known as the Slave or Bottom, a Sub might enjoy the idea of being humiliated, of being told what to do, or of being restrained. The big thing here is submission and penetration go hand in hand—the idea of being taken and penetrated can be extremely arousing to a Submissive. Some Subs expect pleasure in return, while, for other Submissives, the only goal is to pleasure their Doms.

Switch It Up

Some people are only comfortable in one of the roles—Dom or Sub—while others can assume either role, depending on the mood or setting. These are the same versatile folks who do well at large parties and small gatherings, who don't mind driving or being in the passenger seat, or who can watch super-dude action films and chick flicks. If you're just getting started, try several different role-play scenarios and see where you feel most comfortable.

That's the beauty of BDSM, it's a fascinating way to explore yourself and your partner through a perversely intimate power exchange, a way to turn reality upside down and own it on your own terms. The key to making the dynamic work is trust. Yep, BDSM is like one big trust fall.

73. Honest Couples Have the Best Sex

Are you and your partner honest with each other? Do you tell him when you feel safe or how you're feeling about your relationship in general? A big culprit of a low libido is not feeling close to your partner; feeling emotionally distant can really take a toll on your sex life. If you no longer feel emotionally safe with your partner, you may have less and less desire to be sexual with him.

Here's the thing. Most of the time, one partner doesn't even realize that there is a problem. It's important to start talking honestly and opening up to him emotionally, provided he does the same with you. If you're truly having trouble with this, a counselor or therapist can help you and your partner start to see eye to eye.

Once you and your partner become close again emotionally, you'll find that you want to experience each other sexually, as well.

74. Position Yourself for Pleasure: Try Oral with Manual Stimulation

In this position, you need to lie on your back while your partner stimulates your vagina and G-spot with his fingers and your clitoris with his mouth at the same time. This position is a big hit for women because in this position, it's all about the orgasm. Because you're lying on your back and your partner is resting comfortably on the bed, he can focus on what he needs to do and you can focus on enjoying the sensations. The trick with this position is the gradual build up. Your partner needs to start slow, pay attention to your response, and then increase the intensity as needed.

75. Help Him Get Hard

Although you can get off on your own and your man can get you off with penetration, making sure he stays in the game can be an important part of your sex life. According to WebMD, erectile dysfunction affects an estimated 18 million men in the United States alone. Wow! And that's just the number of men who admit to having a problem. Imagine how many guys aren't willing to admit they can't get it up to someone who calls to do a survey. With all the ads on television for erectile dysfunction medications, you'd think we'd all be experts about it by now. But, what causes the condition? Is there a cure that doesn't involve medication?

What Exactly Is Erectile Dysfunction?

Erectile dysfunction (also known as ED and male impotence) is a sexual dysfunction characterized by the inability to develop or maintain an erection of the penis. But what causes it?

Most people don't realize that erectile dysfunction is not necessarily just a simple physical problem. And guess what? Sometimes it's not even a medical problem! If your partner eats unhealthy foods, never exercises, or regularly stresses out, while going to a job he hates, then he's very unlikely to have the multihour erections he may have had back when you two first hooked up.

The real cause of your partner's problems could be physical, psychological, emotional, or even related to his lifestyle. What's worse, any one underlying issue (even a lifestyle issue) can trigger physical problems, which in turn can cause ED—or many other health problems. For example, a significant amount of stress in his everyday life can leave you open and susceptible to all kinds of illnesses, which, in turn, can trigger other problems. The most common physical causes of erectile dysfunction, according to the Mayo Clinic, include:

- Heart disease.
- Clogged blood vessels (atherosclerosis).
- High blood pressure.
- Diabetes.
- Obesity.
- Metabolic syndrome.

Other causes of erectile dysfunction include:

- Certain prescription medications.
- Tobacco use.
- Alcoholism and other forms of drug abuse.
- Treatments for prostate cancer.
- Parkinson's disease.
- Multiple sclerosis.
- Hormonal disorders such as low testosterone (hypogonadism).
- Peyronie's disease.
- Surgeries or injuries that affect the pelvic area or spinal cord.

No matter what is causing your partner's ED, it's important to identify the core underlying issue and treat it.

What Can You Do about Erectile Dysfunction?

The most important first step to take is to consult a doctor, and correctly diagnose the problem. With all the TV ads advertising the blue pill, the purple pill, and all kinds of other well-marketed pills, it's hard to know what you're actually fixing (or breaking).

All that having been said, once you're well informed and have a qualified medical opinion on the cause of your partner's impotence, it's time to do some serious research and figure out what to do about it.

For male impotence, the more frequently prescribed treatments are medications like Viagra and Cialis. But, in addition to medications, there are various natural and herbal supplements for treating (or reversing) impotence, such as Herbal Viagra. Keep an open mind to natural and alternative approaches. For example, if the problem is ultimately caused by an ongoing stressful situation in his everyday life, then maybe it's to both of your advantages to ease that stress. Sure, some supplements, better diet, and possibly even ED medication (whether prescription or herbal) might also help, but in the long run, dealing with the real issue will help you resolve the root cause of the disorder.

Again, it's very important to visit a doctor and get an informed medical opinion of the situation first. But then, be smart and take the time to research and fully understand your options. Don't just blindly follow what one person tells you, even if you paid a lot of money for that office visit. Just remember that one person may also be blindly following what someone else told him!

Viagra 101

Most of us know what Viagra is—that magic little blue pill that can turn a wet noodle into a flag at full mast. But what is Viagra, really? What are the pros and cons of these erectile dysfunction pills that are only growing in popularity? Is Viagra for you? Here's what's up with Viagra.

Viagra Pros

The most obvious pro of that little blue pill is that it can help many men and women reclaim their sex lives. Men who have been suffering from sexual dysfunction can once again experience fulfilling and satisfying sex, and so can their partners. Viagra works by promoting blood flow to the penis, helping it to become and stay erect when sexually stimulated. When taken as prescribed by a doctor, this little blue pill can help your man become and stay more sexually active and have a fulfilling sex life.

Viagra Cons

Just like any medication, Viagra has side effects as well. Here's the scoop. The most common side effects of Viagra include:

- Dizziness.
- Diarrhea.
- Upset stomach.
- Headaches.

More serious side effects include sudden loss of vision (in rare cases) and a prolonged erection, both of which require immediate medical attention. Men who smoke, have high blood pressure, or heart problems need to discuss these issues with their doctors extensively before trying Viagra.

Make Life Changes

Once you have identified what situation in your partner's life may be contributing to impotence, take steps to correct it! If your sex life isn't what it could be, then fix it. There's no good excuse for a miserable sex life. Take steps to rekindle the romance, and spice up your sex life. Talk to your partner about your intentions, and see what you can come up with together to reinvigorate the magic. It can be done, but you have to really want it and make a commitment to it.

And, of course, there's never a bad time to start an exercise program (one that your doctor would approve of), or to start eating healthier. Massage and meditation have also been shown to dramatically reduce stress and help increase your and your partner's quality of life, sex, and otherwise.

76. *Have Hot Sex, Even If Your Kids Are Home*

There's a lot of controversy on this topic. It seems that most people think it's okay to have sex while your kids are home, but only if you're married. Now, if your beliefs require that you only have sex after marriage then that's fine, but today this is rarely the case. The fact is that most people have sex before they're married and it's even more common for subsequent relationships. Having sex while the kids are home is perfectly normal but, obviously, use discretion. Lock the bedroom door!

The job of a parent is not only to provide for her children, but to teach them what a healthy, loving relationship looks like. And a healthy, loving relationship includes sex. Instead of skipping sex when the kids are home and you're in the mood—which will be difficult if they're not yet in school or involved in extracurricular activities—make sex a topic that isn't taboo in the household, but one that is discussed openly with age-appropriate responses when your kids ask you questions. When you know that your children realize that sex is something that happens between two people who love each other, it will make it that much easier for you to have amazing sex—even when they're in the house.

HE **SAYS . . .**

Guess what, if your kids hear you talk about sex, they'll know it's normal and okay to talk about. And if they have questions, they'll ask you instead of the kids at school. Trust me, they *will* have questions and parents who refuse to expose their kids to sexual topics inadvertently push them into learning incorrect facts from their friends. Do you really want your kids to learn about sex from their friends? And do you want them growing up thinking that a normal relationship does not include sex? Think about that.

77. Show Some Skin

This secret is targeted at those of you who have forgotten how to dress sexy—or never really knew how. Go out and buy something truly revealing—low cut, short, tight, clingy, etc. If you can't figure out if what you picked is really lingerie in disguise, you'll know you have the right outfit.

Wear this outfit on your next date. Now, if you're going to a location where the outfit is truly inappropriate, then wear a coat or wrap over it and then take the coat off at some point. If you're going to a restaurant, take the coat off when you sit down. If you're going to a movie, take the coat off once you're inside. You get the idea. Your man will be so excited knowing what's under the coat, that he won't be able to control himself.

HE **SAYS . . .**

Men love to see their woman playing along, showing initiative. Dressing provocatively for him shows him you're interested and encourages him to want and fantasize about you even more. After all, he will fantasize about someone; wouldn't you prefer it be you?

78. *Position Yourself for Pleasure: Try the Deep Stick*

This position is very similar to missionary except your partner is not on top, but is instead kneeling with your legs on his shoulders. This is a great position if your man has a shorter penis because it allows him to penetrate you deeper and stimulate your G-spot or the even deeper A-spot that lies just beyond the cervix which can result in a mind-blowing orgasm. Just be careful and communicate with him if this position becomes painful if he's on the lengthier side. Remember, deeper is not always better.

79. *Enjoy a Clothing-Optional Weekend*

There's no better way to let go of your inhibitions than to run around naked—and not freak out the neighbors. So, the idea here is to check into your favorite hotel or resort away from home and spend the entire weekend naked. It will need to be a hotel with room service because you won't be leaving the room—

at least not with your clothes on. Not only will you discover how to be comfortable in your own skin, it will guarantee that you have sex more often. He simply won't be able to keep his hands off you!

The rules are simple. Once you walk in the door of the hotel room, the clothes must go. You'll be surprised at how good you feel after a few hours. It's very freeing to be completely naked. You may never want to get dressed again.

If you're really feeling adventurous, check into a clothing-optional resort like Desire or Hedonism so that you aren't limited to running around naked only in your room.

80. Get Off More Often

Are you one of those women who really struggles to have orgasms? Are your orgasms few and far between? Well, it's time to solve that problem once and for all.

SexMYTH: Your Orgasms Get Weaker As You Age As you get older, it's important to take care of your body. Eat healthy, exercise, get regular checkups, the whole bit. But, while your hormones will change, it doesn't mean that the sex will go downhill. You may find different things work for you, but you'll still be able to have mind-blowing powerful orgasms.

Almost all women are physically capable of having orgasms, it's just that they can let things like stress, feeling tired, or worrying about all they have to do get in the way. Letting go of all of that will dramatically increase your chances of having an orgasm. Here are a few tips that can help you achieve better, stronger, and more frequent orgasms.

Relax

It is critical for you to take the time you need to transition from a stressful day of work, kids, and household chores to reaching orgasm. If your mind is reeling from all the things you have to do, if you are too tired, or worried, it's probably not going to happen.

Take a bath or shower, enjoy a massage or cup of tea—do whatever you need to do to let go of all the activity in your mind and just relax.

HE **SAYS . . .**

Guys love it when you let loose. Seeing a girl totally let go during sex is a very erotic bonding experience. This is *not* a bad thing; trust yourself and your partner and you'll be closer—and have better sex—for it.

Warm Up

Women need warm-up time and lots of it.

Gradually ease into your sexual self rather than trying to rush and fit a quickie into your already hectic day. Take the time to enjoy an activity that you find sexually stimulating. Warm-up for you could be anything from reading a steamy romance novel to twenty minutes of oral sex. Experiment with your partner to find out what turns you on most.

Let Go

This is where it gets challenging for most women. When things start to feel really good, many women tense up. We're so used to being in charge, that we try to control our orgasms rather than releasing into them—and that's a recipe for disaster.

Women can also tend to be self-conscious about their bodies, or making too much noise, but to experience amazing orgasms, you have to just let go. Yes, that means accepting that belly roll, loving your cellulite, and not being afraid to release those guttural noises that you've been holding in. If your man knows that you're excited, he won't care about anything else!

81. *Lose Your Panties for a Good Time*

Wearing silky lingerie under your clothes can feel really sexy, but going completed naked under there can be incredibly arousing for both you and your partner! A great way to release your inhibitions is to wear a loose-fitting clinging dress for the day with absolutely nothing under it; this is especially true if you choose clothing made from a soft, silky fabric. The feel of the fabric on your nipples and the wind blowing up your skirt will have you squirming with excitement in no time. Your partner will be able to think of nothing but the fact that you are completely naked under that dress. Not to mention the fact that it would be so easy for him to just pull up the skirt and take you. It will be a challenge to not have hot sex!

82. *Spice Things Up for Long-Term Fun*

Relationships (even new ones) require effort. And that includes putting the effort in to keep things interesting in the bedroom. You want to experience your partner intimately and of course, your partner wants to experience you that way too! If you've lost interest in sex, don't fret. You can find it again and with a little work, you can be back on track to having the best sex of your life.

Physical Reasons

There are plenty of reasons a woman can lose interest in having sex with her partner. One of those reasons might be physical. If you're on any medications, research their side effects. For instance, antidepressants and, ironically, birth control pills can diminish your sex drive so you may want to talk with your doctor to see if you can switch types as another may not have the same effect.

If you aren't on medications and you still wonder if the problem is physical, ask your doctor to determine if you have a hormonal imbalance. Sometimes, a low level of testosterone can cause disinterest in sexual activity and high levels of estrogen can do the same. Your doctor may be able to recommend solutions so you can once again have a fulfilling sex life.

*Sex*MYTH: **All Men Love Lingerie** If your boyfriend or husband always steals the lingerie catalog when it shows up at your house, it's probably not the lingerie he's enjoying as he flips from page to page. It's the nearly naked models. Because while some men are into push-up bras or garter belts or corsets, other guys just want you naked as fast as possible so they can enjoy looking at your body. If you want to purchase sexy lingerie to make yourself feel good, by all means, do. But if you're buying it to turn him on, make sure he'll appreciate it before spending the Benjamins.

Emotional Reasons

Relationship bumps can also make you feel less interested in sex. But, if sometimes the problems go deeper—perhaps stemming from trauma that happened at another time in your life—they can have a negative impact on your current relationship and your interest in sex. If this is the case for you, it might be worth making an appointment with a professional so that you can start healing your emotional self and learn to enjoy sex once again. By giving you the tools you need, you can push past these emotional issues and get your sex life headed to where you want it to be.

HE **SAYS** . . .

We get so busy with life, especially after having kids, that sometimes a sexual relationship becomes more like one between two buddies. Don't forget the person you fell in love with. We all want to get off, sometimes we just need to be reminded of how much we need it.

Life Balance

Are you running on fumes? Not getting a full eight hours of sleep? Not taking any time for yourself? Then we're not surprised your interest in sex has waned. You're expending so much energy throughout the day without taking the time to recharge that it's no wonder you don't have any left over for sex. Schedule some alone time for yourself every day, even if it's only a half hour. Do something you love, whether it's hitting the gym or working on your knitting. And, for goodness sake, turn off your cell phone during this time so you can fully disconnect from everything that might be causing you stress. It's also worth it to work together with your partner to make these changes so that he can do the same in his life, leaving you both the energy to experience each other sexually.

Discord with Your Partner

Sometimes sexual disinterest occurs if you don't feel emotionally safe with or connected to your partner. Contrary to popular belief, sex and intimacy have everything to do with feeling emotionally connected and safe with someone.

If you don't feel connected and safe, it's likely that you're not going to be interested in sharing yourself sexually. You can help bring your relationship together so you can have a better sex life by doing a number of things. For example, if your relationship is really distant, you can consider seeing a relationship counselor or a therapist. You can also start by talking to your partner and sharing your life with him. Take time out of your day for each other! You'd be surprised at how many men and women feel like they are roommates rather than partners after awhile. Sharing a life together is something that can really help bring you together sexually later on.

83. Sex Toys Provide Variety

Sex toys come in many, many different shapes, sizes, colors, and materials. With a little experimentation, you'll find what works for you and you lover. To get you on your way, here's a quick breakdown of the most common toys:

Vibrators

When most people refer to sex toys they're generally thinking of basic vibrators—a simple, mostly straight, phallius-shaped object that happens to also have a built-in vibrating mechanism, but that's just the beginning. There are vibrators for every pleasure!

SexMYTH: Vibrators Replace Men Many men are afraid that a vibrator will give a woman such intense sexual pleasure that she won't desire actual sex anymore, but that's simply not true! There's nothing that replaces the closeness and intimacy of sex with your partner, not even the best and most expensive vibrator.

G-spot Vibrators

We discuss G-spot vibrators in Entry #67, but wanted to go in more depth here. G-spot vibrators are some of the most popular vibrators available. They're curved and when used properly, they can help you reach the ultimate G-spot stimulation! They're fun to use with a partner or just by yourself and can be incorporated into many different types of sex play. Many G-spot vibrators come equipped with clitoral stimulators that can help give you dual pleasure.

Clitoral Vibrators

Many women can only achieve orgasm through clitoral stimulation, which makes clitoral vibrators very popular. They can be used with or without a partner, and there are many types of clitoral vibrators—from the small and discreet bullet to the extreme sensations of the Hitachi Magic Wand—that can be used during sex to provide heightened pleasure. Many are available in waterproof versions and most of them can fit almost any budget.

Discreet Vibrators

Many women prefer to use smaller, discreet vibrators that cannot easily be distinguished from other everyday items. Sometimes the larger vibrators can be a bit intimidating and difficult to store in discreet way. We've all heard the story of the woman's vibrator falling out of her suitcase at the airport. Well, discreet vibrators are small enough that they easily fit in a purse or a pocketbook and can be disguised as a lighter, a tube of lipstick, or other types of everyday items and if the kids find it, you can just say that it's your really cool new USB drive for your computer. Plus, they're economical and, contrary to popular belief, the right discreet vibrator can pack quite a punch.

Finger Vibrators

Finger vibrators are exactly what they sound like, vibrators that fit right onto your finger! While many couples use finger vibrators together, they're great for female masturbation because they work well with the way a woman naturally masturbates. Some finger vibrators can be expensive, but many can be found at a good price.

Remote, Bullet, and Egg Vibrators

While you can use a remote vibrator by yourself, they are best shared with a partner; it can be really fun to put your pleasure in someone else's hands! Just imagine your partner being able to give you a buzz whenever he feels like it. These are really good for some of those domination/submission games we talked about in Entry #72. You can be his sex slave and when he buzzes, you absolutely must 'come.'

You can also give bullet or egg vibrators a try. These vibrators are small, discreet, and provide comfort, versatility, and intense pleasure. Bullets are very popular for these reasons, but they are not intended for insertion into your vagina. Egg vibrators, on the other hand, are intended for insertion and can be positioned to provide pleasure directly to your G-spot.

If you're interested in buying a vibrator to use either by yourself or with your partner, there are a multitude of websites that offer the widest variety of vibrators so you can find the one you're looking for. Just remember to have fun and experiment with different vibrators! You might find that you like more than one.

HE **SAYS . . .**

Vibrators aren't just for solo use. Guys want to be involved too. Couples can have a lot of fun by sharing their pleasure with each other by using toys. Keep us involved, you'll be glad you did!

Dildos

Dildos basically look like most people's idea of a vibrator, but they are not motorized. They're entirely hand activated, and are intended for clitoral or vaginal stimulation—although, as is the case with most sex toys, intended use and actual creative use in practice are not always the same. They, of course, also come in many shapes and sizes.

Harnesses

Dildos are great, but they're hand powered which means that you won't have your hands available for other types of fondling and play. A harness is a device that is generally strapped around your waist or hips onto which you can attach your favorite dildo.

If you've ever wondered what it would be like to be a man, to have that kind of control, give the harness a try. And the next time he wants to have anal sex with you simply tell him that you will if he will.

Harnesses are great for men too. Have him wear the harness and penetrate you with a dildo instead of his penis. If you want to help intercourse last longer and try some new sizes and textures, having your partner try a harness is a great idea!

Anal Sex Toys

As the name implies, anal toys are basically dildos designed for anal penetration. The biggest difference between a regular dildo and an anal sex toy is that anal toys have flared ends to prevent them from getting lost. For this very reason you should never use a standard dildo or other sex toy for anal play. Emergency rooms are full of people who used the wrong toys anally. Be sure to stick with toys from a reputable company that are specifically designed for anal insertion to be safe.

Penis Rings

A penis ring (or cock ring) is a rubber or metal ring that's worn around the base of the penis. Penis rings give your partner added pleasure, plus penis rings can sometimes help him maintain a harder erection for longer periods of time. And when erections last longer, sex lasts longer. Sounds like a win-win situation to us!

Homemade Sex Toys

You'll be surprised to discover how many potential sex toys you have floating around your own home. Of course, think twice before you start using your various household objects for sexual play. Consider cleanliness, safety, and whether you still plan to use that spatula for cooking tomorrow.

Here are just a few examples of household items that can be used as sex toys:

- Your back massager—if it's really a back massager in the first place.
- Vegetables—think cucumbers, carrots, zucchini, etc. Just make sure to wash them thoroughly and use a condom over the vegetable to reduce the risk of getting a bacterial infection.
- Satin sheets—they'll feel great rubbed against your clitoris.
- Jets in your whirlpool bath.
- The handle of your electric toothbrush.
- The handle of your favorite spatula or hair brush.

HE **SAYS** . . .

Sex toys aren't just for women. Lots of men—straight, bisexual, or gay—actually enjoy sex toys, including anal toys, cock rings, restraints, and more. Use your imagination and don't limit yourself by common societal stereotypes.

These days you can easily and cheaply obtain sex toys that are specifically designed for safe and enjoyable sex play. That's by far our recommendation from a safety and enjoyment standpoint. Why use a vegetable when you can use a Rabbit?

Restraints and Other Bondage Toys

Sex play of the dominant and submissive variety (BDSM) usually involves various props that fall into the toy category. These toys range from satin restraints, leather-wear, and nipple clamps, to blindfolds, cuffs, mouth gags, and whatever else does it for you.

84. Don't Step Outside the Box

A Fantasy Box is something you can try if you or your partner are really shy about sharing your fantasies. Write down your fantasies on a scrap piece of paper and put it in the box. Have your partner do the same. Make a rule that once a week, a fantasy is pulled out of the box and played out. It's fun to be spontaneous, and both you and your partner already know you'll be acting out a fantasy, so you'll be in a great mindset to have a good time! Some fantasies take a bit of preparation, so it can also be fun to pull a fantasy out of the box a few weeks ahead of time and go shopping together for toys, lubes, or costumes—whatever your fantasy requires! Decorate the fantasy box with things you both find sexy to make it even more fun.

85. Massage His Lingham

What is a *Lingham*? This term for the male penis can be translated as "wand of light." In tantric sex, it represents the Divine Male Sexual Energy and Consciousness. This type of positive language helps bring an emotional connection between partners during sex and helps generate an atmosphere where both lovers feel valued, respected, and nurtured. To help set the scene for this magical experience to take place, think about how to create a warm, relaxing, and seductive environment. Some things you might want to include are:

- Relaxing, seductive music. Preferably something without words or, if that isn't possible, something with words in another language.
- Eye-catching visuals such as luxurious throws or pretty flowers that help frame the cozy space.

- A warm, welcoming space. How can you feel frisky if you don't feel comfortable first?
- Sexy clothes. How you look on the outside can affect how you feel on the inside. Make sure you are thinking sexy, by looking sexy. Your partner will love the way you look, if you feel that way too.

Try to set some time aside for your tantric pleasure experience as a way to honor your lover, develop skills, relax, and focus the mind and spirit.

Giving a Lingham Massage

Before jumping right in to massaging the Lingham, help your partner relax with a luxurious massage that lasts at least thirty minutes. It will help him get used to your touch and move into a sensual space where he can more appreciate a Lingham massage instead of just wanting a hand job.

Drip warm vegetable, organic, or cold-pressed oil over the Lingham, scrotum, and perineum (a small circular area between the scrotum and anus). Do not use pure or diluted essential oils internally or near intimate areas and avoid oil-based products, instead use only pure, organic vegetable oils such as olive or grape seed oils.

Gently massage up and down the shaft and very lightly at the head. Remember you are slowly building up to a wonderful crescendo, so initially less is more. Massage the scrotum gently, all while getting feedback from him about the pressure he prefers.

The perineum is referred to as the *Sacred Spot* by Tantrists and is a great place to give him some incredible sensations. This is a very sensitive area, so apply only gentle pressure using the tips of your finger in a circular motion for a few minutes at a time.

Increase the pressure of your strokes over and along the Lingham, and massage the head by twisting your hand in a left-right direction. If his sensations become too intense, stop, slow down, and encourage him to take some slow deep breaths.

The slow, luxurious-release approach of intimate tantric massage is always a welcome indulgence. So lavish the Lingham with pure sensuality and divine love and attention. Your lover is likely to reciprocate.

86. *Position Yourself for Pleasure: Try Spooning*

Spooning is a position to try first thing in the morning—or in the middle of the night. To get into the spooning position, your partner needs to lie on his side behind you in the Spooning cuddle position—only he'll penetrate you from behind rather than simply snuggling. This position works great for either vaginal or anal sex. Your breasts are easily accessible as are the sensitive areas on the back of your neck and ears. Plus this position is very intimate and the penetration angle is great for G-spot and clitoral stimulation. He's also not supporting all of his weight, so he'll be able to go longer (physically at least). This may very well be the perfect sex position!

87. *Don't Forget to Have Fun*

When you start dating someone, everything is fun. Just holding his hand can be a rush. But, eventually, the novelty fades. To make a relationship last and to make the sex more spontaneous and enjoyable, it's important to remind each other about why you two got together in the first place by keeping the fun alive. Remember, if you're able to let loose, kick back, and just focus on having a great time, the sex is apt to be amazing

Sex MYTH: Women Shouldn't Have Fun During Sex Says who? Though society used to have the idea that women only had sex to please their men and to be able to have children, times have changed. If you're still living under that idea, it's time to start taking the reins in bed and making sure he is satisfying you as much as he is pleasuring himself. If he's not the type to get on board with this, consider finding a man who will!

Act Like Kids

Sometimes, as adults, it's easy to fall into a routine where dates involve dinner and a movie and life can get a little too serious. At these times, it's important to break out of the rut and plan some events with your partner when you can both just let loose and have fun. Whether that means a trip to the amusement park or making a snowman and throwing snowballs at each other, returning to a state of childlike wonder and fun can bring back the joy and playfulness that led to really great sex when you and your partner first got together.

Be Silly . . . In Bed

You might not have thought about this, but it's okay to be funny in bed. After all, sex is kind of funny on its own. Whether it's the noises your bodies make when you're making love or the strange appearance of our sex organs, sex doesn't have to always be serious. It can be lighthearted. When you're not in the middle of a super romantic moment, consider tickling your partner or just being goofy and giving him a raspberry. By being playful, it can bring the two of you closer together and more apt to enjoy life with each other outside of the bedroom too. And the happier the relationship and the more in sync you and your partner are, the higher the likelihood that you will have amazing sex.

HE **SAYS . . .**

Please don't fake orgasms. From a man's standpoint that's just being untruthful. You're doing both yourself and your man a disservice.

88. *Know When the "O" Shows Up*

If you ask a group of women to describe their orgasms, you're likely to get as many different descriptions as the number of women that you speak with. But all of them will tell you this: When you have an orgasm, you'll know it. It could be as subtle as a tiny shiver up your spine or strong enough to make your whole body shake, but nothing feels quite the same as having an orgasm. And while not all sex has to involve orgasms, you won't be able to experience great sex without having them. If you're not sure that you've been having orgasms—and sometimes women have a hard time reaching orgasm during sex or with a new partner—focus on having intense orgasms on your own. Hone your masturbation techniques until you're sure you are making yourself come, then take what works for you when you're pleasuring yourself and adapt it to work with your partner. Once you know what a great orgasm feels like, you'll know what to aim for when you're with someone else, which will only lead to better and better sex.

89. *Eat and Drink to Feel Sexy*

While this is not a book on nutrition, there are a few things that you need to know about how what you eat affects your sex drive. Eating a healthy diet and drinking plenty of water are critical to your overall health and well-being, but did you realize that they also have the potential to boost your libido?

People who eat healthy, well-balanced diets containing lots of raw fruits and vegetables, complex carbohydrates, and high-quality proteins naturally have more energy and higher libidos than people who eat poor diets high in fats and processed carbohydrates. Just pay attention to how you feel after you eat a large plate of pasta. You barely want to move, much less have sex!

Below there are some lists of foods that are reported to increase energy and/or libido. Try to incorporate as many of them as possible into your diet on a regular basis, but be careful. While many foods, vitamins, and minerals are reported to increase libido, many of them do not have the stamp of approval from the FDA for this purpose, so you should always consult your doctor or qualified herbalist before starting any type of libido-enhancement plan.

Fiery Foods

Warming and aromatic foods help to energize the body's fire energy and many of them are reported to have other healing properties as well.

These fiery foods include:

- Anise
- Black pepper
- Cardamom
- Cayenne pepper
- Chives
- Cinnamon
- Fennel
- Ginger
- Horseradish
- Leeks
- Onion
- Scallion
- Turmeric

HE **SAYS . . .**

It's hard to know what will and what won't boost the libido in any one individual. Do your best to generally eat light, frequent meals and enjoy healthy foods (particularly fruits and vegetables). And avoid chemicals / preservatives and processed foods as much as possible; you'll feel much better for it.

Essential Omegas

Foods high in essential omega fatty acids are also reported to increase libido. Both cold-water and deep-sea fish are included on this list:

- Halibut
- Salmon
- Sardines

Miscellaneous Others

Here are some other foods that are said to increase libido:

- **Almonds:** Good source of essential fatty acids. Always choose raw almonds (and other nuts). The roasting process reduces the nutritional value of nuts.
- **Avocado:** Contain high levels of folic acid, B6, and potassium. B6 is reported to increase male hormone production and potassium helps to regulate a woman's thyroid gland.
- **Bananas:** Contain potassium, B vitamins, and riboflavin which all help increase the body's energy levels. Plus, bananas also contain bromelain, an enzyme reported to increase libido.
- **Celery:** Contains a similar hormone to what is released through male perspiration. Don't worry, it's odorless.
- **Chocolate:** Contains theobromine, which is a compound similar to caffeine. Dark chocolate (which has a higher cocoa concentration) also contains phenylethylamine, an amino acid that enhances your mood.
- **Eggs:** High in vitamins B6 and B5.
- **Figs:** High in amino acids.
- **Garlic:** In addition to being aromatic and warming, garlic contains allicin, which is reported to increase blood flow to the sexual organs.
- **Liver:** Good source of glutamine.
- **Raw Oysters:** Oysters deserve a mention because they are the most commonly noted aphrodisiac. Is it because they are high in zinc and contain dopamine? Or is it the erotic act of sucking the oyster from the shell that's the real turn-on? Give them a try and find out for yourself.

90. *Be a Little Uptight*

Creams, supplements, and even equipment for penis enlargement or erectile dysfunction are readily available for men all over the world, but what about what women want? It's true, after childbirth and as women age, the vagina can become loose and lose sensitivity for both partners. What's a gal to do when having sex just isn't as pleasurable as it used to be? Thankfully, you have a few options that will help get you back in the saddle.

Vaginoplasty

One of the options for vaginal rejuvenation is vaginoplasty, or vaginal surgery. Experienced surgeons can help tighten things up down south, giving you and your partner a more satisfying sex life—but is vaginal surgery all it's cracked up to be? Not exactly. As with any surgery, while there are pros, there is also a long list of cons. The worst being death, followed by infection, undesirable results (such as a vagina that is still too loose or becomes too tight to even have intercourse), and a long recovery period even if the surgery goes off without a hitch. Any woman considering vaginoplasty should talk to a board-certified surgeon and consider all options before consenting to surgery.

Are There Other Options?

Of course! The most tried and true of all of them are the well-known Kegel exercises. You may have heard of them, but might not ever have tried them. You can try doing Kegels on their own, or you take it up a notch by using vaginal weights or Ben-Wa balls. Check out Entry #41 to learn more!

Another option is vaginal tightening cream. Just like anti-wrinkle cream for your face, vaginal tightening cream claims to plump and hydrate the inner walls of the vagina, giving you and your partner heightened sensitivity during sex. Combined with Kegel exercises, vaginal tightening cream may help produce even better results than vaginal surgery, without the risks and lengthy healing period.

Before considering vaginoplasty, you should first exhaust all other options. Through discovering different ways to tighten and tone your vaginal tissue and muscles, you can bring the passion back to your sex life without expensive and risky vaginal surgery.

91. *Get Away from It All*

This may seem like a no-brainer, but take a vacation together, just you and your partner. This should not be one of those see-everything, do-everything vacations where you're so exhausted when you get home that you need a vacation to recover from your vacation. This is time to nurture the relationship.

HE **SAYS . . .**

We absolutely love to take three or four day weekends at our local Four Seasons resort as often as we can get away (ideally every month or two). It's a sort of home away from home where we can go and focus on time together, not worry about the chores, things that need cleaning or fixing, work, or anything else for that matter. A regular romantic change of venue can be just what the doctor ordered.

It doesn't matter if it's a weekend, a week, or a month, but check yourselves into a hotel or take a cruise where the only activity you schedule is spending time together and having fun. Nothing works to spice up your sex life more than a little time away from home.

92. *Tantric Sex Gets You Off Over and Over Again*

While multiple orgasms seem like an unattainable goal that should be something talked about only in sex myths, they really are attainable. By following some tantric practices, you'll have an easier time achieving multiple orgasms even if you've had a hard time doing so in the past. By harnessing the powerful energies flowing through your body, you and your partner can connect to each other's sexual energies and open pathways that allow this energy to flow more freely and more effectively between you two, so it is easier to reach the peak of ecstasy.

Just Breathe

If you're still doubtful that you can have multiple orgasms, or if you think they're too complicated for you to figure out, try this difficult step first: Breathe. How hard was that? Exactly. A lot of tantra involves connecting your spiritual self to your physical and emotional self, and that involves deep breathing and inner peace. Through breath, the followers of tantra believe that you can clear blocked chakras that have been holding you back. Through controlled breathing, you can establish a physical connection with your partner that will help you climax over and over and over, and may even lead to simultaneous multiple orgasms.

Like everything, breathing properly requires practice. "But," you say, "I already know how to breathe!" Well, of course you do, or you probably wouldn't be reading this book. But deep, controlled breathing is different and as you may have already realized, it isn't easy to control your breathing during the throes of sex. But the following primary exercises can help you get a handle on the basic concept.

Primary Breathing Exercise

Take a deep breath in through your nose, pushing out your stomach as you do so. Then breathe out slowly through your mouth. Don't breathe in or out so much the air is forced or the breathing feels uncomfortable. The goal here is for the breath to relax you and help you let go of any stress you're holding onto. As you get the hang of the slower movement, you can try doing it rapidly as this will have an energizing effect and be more useful during sexual play.

Put It into Practice

Now that you and your partner both understand how to breathe to both relax and energize yourselves, try doing it together. Once in bed, synchronize your breathing so that your energies are on the same level. Then begin exchanging air with him so that as he breathes out, you'll breathe in and vice versa. As you connect with your partner, you may even find it's easy to achieve not just one, but multiple orgasms.

No Pressure

When you're on your journey to have more than one orgasm try not to make that the goal. Instead, focus on having fun and connecting with your partner. As you explore each other and appreciate him more on a physical and spiritual level, the orgasms will follow naturally.

Releasing the Female Orgasm

For women, the quality of the sex has a lot to do with what is going on in the brain. You don't want to let fear, guilt, stress, or other distracting thoughts get in the way of getting off, but sometimes, it's hard to stop thoughts about what's for dinner, how much work you have left to do for the night, or anything else, from crowding in and taking over. When this happens, switch up the action and pleasure your partner or ask him to pleasure you so you're able to be distracted enough to bring the focus back on what you're feeling sexually, and off of those lingering thoughts.

HE **SAYS . . .**

Believe it or not, one of a man's primary goals in bed is to satisfy the woman he's with. We get great pleasure from helping our partner reach orgasm and when we manage to make her experience multiple orgasms, it is a huge turn-on and a confidence booster because it means we're doing an incredible job. And that just makes us want to have even more sex!

One great way to distract yourself is to ask him to pay special attention to your clitoris. As he stimulates the clitoris and labia with his fingers and tongue, respond with sounds to signal to him when he's in the right spot. You'll soon find your focus has been shifted to the throbbing pleasure you're feeling down below.

Guide Him on His Way

To help him out, make sure he pays ample attention to your G-spot or *sacred spot* as it is referred to in tantra. It is located two to three inches inside the vagina on the side that faces your navel, and when stimulated can cause intense orgasms and, in some women, ejaculation.

93. Sufficient Sleep Leads to Hot Sex

Lack of sleep and being tired are some of the major reasons that a woman may not be able to orgasm or to even get aroused. According to SleepWeb.com (*www.sleepweb.com*), lack of sleep seriously affects your sex drive. It:

- Can make you moody, stressed, or anxious and, as result, less likely to be eager for sex.
- Slows the basic thought processes. If you're not thinking straight, you may say or do something that can ruin the moment. Sleeplessness makes you less mentally aware. When your brain isn't processing as fast as it could be, you might inadvertently do something that derails the train to great sex.
- Causes drowsiness. No surprise there, but falling asleep during sex doesn't usually lead to a good time for either party.

We all need different amounts of sleep. Some get by just fine on 6–7 hours of sleep, while others need at least 8–9 hours of sleep every night. Sleep is the time in which our body heals and repairs itself. So, get to bed early! It's critical that women (and men) arrange their schedules and activities so that they are getting enough sleep—and enough sex.

94. *Position Yourself for Pleasure: Do It Doggie Style*

Doggie Style is the second most common sexual position in the United States. In this position, you'll be on all fours with your partner penetrating you from behind. While not the most intimate position, this is a great position for hitting the G-spot and it's very easy for your man to reach around and stimulate your clitoris.

*Sex*MYTH: **Not All Women Have a G-Spot** So not true. While not all women have an easy time finding their G-spots or like having their G-spots pleasured, all women have one. If you're having trouble finding yours, consider investing in a G-spot dildo that is designed in such a way to make it easy to pinpoint this small area.

This is another position where neither of you have to support all of your weight so you'll be able to last longer physically. Many times women give out physically before they are able to orgasm, especially when doing some of the more challenging sexual positions. Doggie Style and other positions like this greatly increase your chances of being able to relax into orgasm rather than focusing on keeping your balance or rhythm. It's also one of the most flexible positions because you can do it standing up, leaning over, or on all fours and it's easy to switch between the options until you find the angle you like the most.

95. Talk about Your Troubles

Men and women communicate very differently. When it comes to the touchy topic of sex, men tend to talk too little and women tend to talk too much.

You may want to hash out the details in a very matter of fact way, but this approach will make a man run for the hills every time. He will become defensive which, in turn, will cause you to feel frustrated; this normally results in nothing getting solved and with everyone feeling at least a little bitter about how the conversation did or didn't go.

Your man may have a very difficult time sharing his feelings, and talking about sex with you may feel like the equivalent to shoving a splinter under his fingernails. The sooner you accept that he doesn't want to talk about sex or how he's doing in bed, the better it will be for both of you.

HE **SAYS . . .**

Whatever you do, don't ever tell your guy anything that sounds in any way like "we need to talk." That just makes us think of the worst-case scenario, so don't do it! If your partner thinks you're about to break up with him, he is *not* going to be mentally and emotionally open to suggestions.

That doesn't mean that you shouldn't talk about sex, however. You need to be completely honest with each other about everything that happens in your relationship and that includes talking about how your sex life is going. Just recognize that these conversations are difficult for him and try to make the conversations flow more smoothly. After all, once he knows what's wrong in the bedroom, he'll do everything in his power to make it right.

96. *Buy Sex Toys in Secret*

The good news is that buying a sex toy today means having more options than ever before. (Read more about the perks in Entry #83.) You can buy sex toys in person or online from a variety of different stores—drugstores, lingerie stores, adult video stores, and of course novelty stores. The benefit of shopping in person is that you can get a better idea for the actual size and shape of the sex toy as well as the weight and feel. Plus, the individuals working in the store normally know a lot about the toys and can help you choose the right toy for you.

But sometimes, it can be a turn-on to buy items over the Internet. Because when that discreet package is delivered right to your door or to your office, you'll know just what's inside and get an extra kick out of the fact that no one is the wiser. And if your partner is there and accidentally opens it before you get home, you might just be in for a pleasant surprise.

97. *Break a Sweat for Better Sex*

Physical activity has been clinically proven to improve sexual health. Just thirty minutes of exercise every day can dramatically improve your health, increase your energy levels, and even increase your libido.

You don't have to spend hours in the gym, in fact you don't even have to go to the gym. It doesn't matter what you do, just do something—walking, jogging, swimming, cycling, strength training, yoga, tae kwon do (or another martial art), or dancing, the list goes on and on. The point is to just get moving. Make it a goal to break a sweat every day.

98. Position Yourself for Pleasure: Try the Modified Missionary

The Missionary position is one of the most common—and probably the most frequently used—sexual positions. It's definitely one of the most simple and most intimate. Basically, you lie on your back and your partner lies on top of you for penetration. However, basic Missionary is not the first choice for pleasure unless you add a few simple modifications.

- **Modification #1:** Have him bring your bent knees up under his shoulders, or if you are flexible enough, over his shoulders. This will allow for much better G-spot stimulation.
- **Modification #2:** Have him hold your legs in a V shape. This will provide a little more space for either you or your partner to stimulate your clitoris.

99. Safe Makes It Sexy

We discussed different types of contraception in Entry #66, but we wanted to go into more detail about the benefits of safe sex here. There is nothing that makes sex better than knowing that you're not going to get pregnant and that you're not going to catch something you'd rather not. Sex is best when you are relaxed, so make sure it's safe and have fun!

Sexually Transmitted Diseases (STDs)

STDs, as their name states, are diseases that are transferred during sex. And in this case, oral, vaginal, and anal sex count. The best way to protect yourself from STDs is by using a dental dam during cunnilingus and a condom during fellatio and when having either vaginal or anal sex (switch condoms if you go from anal to vaginal to prevent bacteria from spreading). When you use condoms and dental dams, you can still explore each other sexually and you can do so without the risk of catching a disease, making sex that much more free and fun. If you want to learn more about specific diseases, read the information on legitimate websites, such as WebMD (*www.webmd.com*) or the Centers for Disease Control (CDC) website (*www.cdc.gov*) and be well informed. After all, smart women are sexy!

When it comes to sexual activity, it can sometimes be confusing to figure out what can spread STDs and what can't. What types of STDs can be contracted during which kinds of sexual activity and when are you completely safe?

There's a reason they're called STDs. You can contract them through virtually any type of sexual activity, including oral sex, anal sex, and vaginal intercourse. But what kinds of STDs are out there and how can you protect yourself?

HIV-AIDS, and Hepatitis C

HIV-AIDS and hepatitis C can be spread via blood-to-blood contact or through vaginal and penile secretions, including semen and pre-cum. The best way to protect yourself against these types of STDs is to use condoms and dental dams while having oral sex, anal sex, and vaginal intercourse. That said, there can always be exceptions and freak occurrences, but the above covers most circumstances.

Other Types of STDs

Other types of STDs include genital herpes and genital warts and are more difficult to protect against. As these types of STDs can actually live in the pubic area of the genitals, a condom or a dental dam may not be enough to protect yourself from contracting one.

This is where STD testing comes in handy. A regular doctor's exam can rule out any of these types of infections. Don't have sexual contact with someone who is experiencing an outbreak of genital herpes or genital warts and don't have sexual contact with anyone who appears to have any type of sores on their genitals.

If you are worried about contracting STDs, it is important to take as many steps toward safety as you can. Regularly get tested for STDs and make sure you wear condoms and use dental dams when having sex. If performing erotic massage, you can wear latex or vinyl gloves and if you decide to try anal sex or rimming, you can use a dental dam or a square of saran wrap. Know who you're with and who they've been with and always be aware of what you're doing. If you're smart and safe, you can significantly reduce your risk of contracting STDs—and being STD-free is sexy.

Can I Get STDs from Masturbation?

The short answer is no. Masturbation is a great pleasure for both men and women. And by masturbating, you can relieve stress and satisfy your sexual desires without having intercourse with someone else. And as long as you don't share your sex toys with anyone else and you wash your hands with soap and water prior to touching yourself (this is a good idea in general, since if you think back to what your hands have touched since you last washed them you probably wouldn't want those same things touching you down below), you should be okay. If you do choose to share your toys with someone else, ask them to use a condom and make sure to wash them with soap and water before you use them again. So go ahead, masturbate to your heart's content and figure out what you like so you can use it in bed the next time you're with someone else!

Oral Sex and STDs: What You Need to Know

It may come as a surprise, but you can catch an STD through oral sex. Though the risk is lower, if you're not in a monogamous relationship in which both partners have been thoroughly tested for STDs, protect yourself during sexual activity of any kind. You can use dental dams, flavored condoms, or even plastic wrap in a pinch! Don't like the way it feels? Try using a little bit of lube on the inside of whatever you choose to create a more natural feeling.

Will This Keep Me Safe?

Unfortunately, even birth control methods that you would think would keep you safe may not be enough to protect you from STDs.

Hormonal Birth Control

While hormonal birth control—commonly referred to as *the pill*—is very effective against preventing pregnancy when taken correctly, it doesn't protect against STDs. Not even one. So, while the sensation of feeling nothing between you and your partner can certainly be sexy . . . consider his sexual history, the seriousness of your relationship, his ability to be faithful, and definitely make sure you and your partner are tested before deciding to rely on this type of contraceptive alone.

Condoms Aren't Always Enough

A little bit of bad news here . . . while condoms and dental dams do protect against most STDs, others—especially herpes and genital warts—can be transmitted even if you're using protection. A regular doctor's exam can rule out any of these types of infections.

However you protect yourself or whoever you're sharing your bed with, make sure any sex you have is safe sex. After all, if you don't have to worry about whether or not you'll catch something by going down on or sleeping with your partner, you can work to give him the best sex possible and, in return, he'll work hard to pleasure you!

100. Come Again

It seems that everyone is talking about multiple orgasms these days. While it's physically possible for almost all women to have multiple orgasms, for some, it's nearly impossible. What makes it so easy for some and impossible for others? Let's start by understanding what we mean by multiple orgasms.

What Is a Multiple Orgasm?

Multiple orgasms simply mean having multiple orgasmic experiences in the same sex session. Unlike your man, you can have another orgasm very quickly after your first, usually within a few seconds or minutes. You don't need the requisite down time that a man needs before he can be aroused again. All women are physiologically able to get off more than once in a row and if you're interested, you can actually train yourself to have multiple orgasms. Here are some tips that will improve your chances of having multiple orgasms:

1. **Learn your body.** Get to know your body and what really turns you on. Once you can easily give yourself one orgasm, you can move on to multiples.

2. **Practice makes perfect.** It takes practice and patience to achieve multiple orgasms. Relax and take as much time as you need. This isn't a race. It's supposed to feel good. Slow down when you need to (even take a break), use lots of lube, and focus on clitoral and G-spot stimulation.

3. **Make sure you're well rested.** What many women don't realize is that being too tired is one of the biggest deterrents to having even one orgasm, much less two or more. If you're well rested, your chances of success are much higher.

4. **Keep going.** After the first orgasm, many women feel quite relaxed and content. It's far too easy to just roll over and go to sleep. Resist the temptation! While it may take 10–15 minutes to reach your first orgasm, the second—and maybe third or fourth—orgasm will come much faster, in just a

few minutes. Don't make yourself exhausted, but keep going as long as you're having fun.

What Is Female Ejaculation?

Basically, when a woman's G-spot is directly stimulated, it can cause a female ejaculatory orgasm, or an expulsion of fluid from the urethra. This fluid is not urine, but a liquid produced and released from the paraurethral glands surrounding the urethra. When these glands are stimulated during intercourse, clitoral stimulation, or most commonly through G-spot stimulation, contractions occur in and around the vagina that cause the fluid to be expelled.

The secret to having G-spot orgasms is to relax and let go. Many women feel like they need to pee just before they have an orgasm, so they hold back. To have a G-spot orgasm, especially one powerful enough to squirt requires that you completely let go—just like during childbirth—and go with the contractions rather than trying to hold them back.

101. Happy, Healthy Women Have the Hottest Sex

Here's a little-known fact. It is impossible to have amazing sex if you're not healthy, happy, and totally in love with yourself. Remember, the secret to incredible, amazing, mind-blowing sex is knowing your body, knowing what you want, knowing how to pleasure yourself, and then having the confidence to share that with your partner. How can you do this if you're miserable, tired, and sick all the time? Take care of yourself spiritually, physically, and emotionally so you can "take care" of yourself in the bedroom. Here are five ways to keep yourself in top sexual form:

1. **Get enough rest.** If you need more sleep than your partner, get the sleep that you need. Having a huge sleep deficit will eventually catch up with you in the form of crankiness, irritability, weight gain or loss, and eventually illness. Life will wait; get the rest you need.

2. **Get a massage.** Massage releases all of the tension and stress stored in your muscles, stimulates blood flow, and simply feels incredible.

3. **Get some sunshine.** Sun exposure is a natural aphrodisiac and moderate sun exposure has many other proven health benefits.

4. **Take a warm bath.** Put a sign on the bathroom door that says "Off-Duty" or "Do Not Disturb" and relax in a hot bath. It's a great transition from a busy day to a romantic evening.

5. **Eat healthy.** Pass on the pizza just for today. Especially if you have a date later in the evening, make sure to eat light; you'll actually feel lighter and have more energy.

Appendix A

Recommended Resources

Online Resources

The following list includes online resources that we can personally recommend to have excellent information on sexuality and improving your sex life.

www.1tantra.com

If what we've written in this guide has sparked your interest in tantra, check out Carla Tara's site where she explores tantra more deeply and helps newcomers to the art understand it using clear and down-to-earth language.

www.adameve.com

When you're looking for sex toys, this is a great resource. Adam & Eve is America's oldest sex toy company and they have a wealth of toys and videos that range from the tame to the super wild. We want to help you on your way toward having mind-blowing sex, so use the offer code "DanJenn" when you check out and save 50 percent on your order.

www.askdanandjennifer.com

We think this site is great. Of course, we're a little biased, because it's ours! Check out our advice column, our online magazine, and our Love & Sex Web show for more tips and advice on how to have the best sex of your life. Plus, the site is also a great place to learn from others in our relationship-support community and share your own knowledge.

www.edenfantasys.com

Eden Fantasys is another great online store that not only offers toys, books, and other products, but also has an online community that you can interact with and learn from.

www.ehow.com

If you're looking for specific tips on something sex or relationship related, check out eHow's library of articles written by both experts and the general online community to find helpful answers. With over 1 million articles and 170,000 high-quality videos, you're likely to find an answer to that burning question of yours.

www.erotic-massage-guide.com

Sometimes, giving an erotic massage can be tricky. Maybe it leads too quickly into sex or your partner becomes so relaxed he falls asleep. For suggestions on how to better harness your massage skills—and learn more about tantra if you so desire—check out Maya Silverman and Guido Harris's in-depth site.

www.healthcentral.com

If you have a sex-related health question or you want to know more about a condition that may be preventing you from having truly enjoyable sex, go to HealthCentral where you can learn from vetted experts and people like you and read real-life health-related experiences and learn information.

http://health.discovery.com

The Discovery Channel has always provided quality scientific content and they don't disappoint with their health information. Find out more about health issues and learn the latest science news and interesting sex facts on this website.

www.idealrelationships.com

If you're having relationship troubles—especially if you're a daddy's girl or your man is a mama's boy—life coaches Joseph and Sarah Elizabeth Malinak want to help.

www.personalchanges.com

Paul Carlson, another life coach, wants to help his clients find happiness, health, and personal wealth on their life journeys. If you think you're in need of some redirecting—be it in your sex life, your relationship, or anything else—you might want to consider giving him a call.

www.sexinfo101.com

Confused about a sex position? Interested in trying something complicated, but not really sure how to maneuver your body? This is one of our absolute favorite websites because it shows more than 100 3D-animated sex positions. Sex positions explained and demonstrated like never seen before. It is jaw-droppingly exciting, inspiring, and totally comprehensive!

http://sexuality.about.com

If you want straight talk on all things sex, look to About.com's sexuality guide Cory Silverberg. He's a certified sexuality educator and he provides friendly, nonjudgmental, and accessible information, encouragement, and advice that will get you to think about sex in different ways.

www.sexuality.org/book

If you can't find what you're looking for, this is a terrific online book that covers all aspects of sexuality in an open and nonjudgmental way.

www.sheknows.com

Getting to the heart of what it really means to be a woman, SheKnows' editors are dedicated to providing daily content for women seeking advice, information, and a fresh, fun take on life—specifically their love life. The SheKnows audience gains access to exclusive content on love, sex, dating, marriage, and all things relationships, as well as beauty, style, entertainment, and more, and are offered a stimulating, well-rounded online experience enhanced with a vibrant message-board community, free games and activities, and captivating blogs.

www.tantra.com

For a closer look into the science and art of tantra and the *Kama Sutra*, this site offers more than 1,000 pages filled with information, lessons, book excerpts, questions and answers, forums, personals, workshop and teacher listings, interviews, videos, e-courses, radio programs, and more. To say it's in-depth would be an understatement.

www.thebeautifulkind.com

Whether you're feeling shy about your sexual desires or have no problem sharing them with the world, this site offers a safe haven for the whole spectrum. It's a sex-positive community where curious minds can gather advice, share their experiences, and learn a thing or two from TBK, a bona fide sex goddess. It's smut for smart people.

www.thisisgreatsex.com

If you're looking for ways to bring love and intimacy back into your relationship, which will certainly help you have great sex, check out this site run by Melody Brooke, a certified marriage and family counselor, author, and speaker. And if you need even more guidance, you can set up a one-hour private phone session with her to help you and your partner work out your issues.

www.webmd.com

This extensive health site was one of the first on the web, and it's a great resource for reference material and anything medically related, including sexual problems.

Printed Resources

The following list includes print resources that we can personally recommend to have excellent information on sexuality and improving your sex life.

The Clitoral Truth by Rebecca Chalker.

This is a very technical but informative book on the female anatomy. You didn't get this information in sex education class. We feel it's a must read for everyone.

The Everything Orgasm Book: The All-You-Need Guide to the Most Satisfying Sex You'll Ever Have by Amy Cooper.

If you want to get off, this is the book for you. Buy it, share it with your man, and clear your calendar because you won't be leaving the bedroom any time soon.

I Love Female Orgasm by Dorian Solot and Marshall Miller.

Complete with stories from both men and women about their favorite positions, worst mistakes, and most amazing moments, this is a book that discusses all parts—and types—of female orgasm.

The One Hour Orgasm by Leah and Bob Schwartz.

This is a very interesting book, but make sure you've got all night to implement the techniques (especially check out the Venus Butterfly technique).

Oral Sex He'll Never Forget: 52 Positions and Techniques Guaranteed to Blow Your Man Away by Sonia Borg, PhD.

This book pretty much does what it says. If you want to give better head, this book will help you master the art of the blow job.

She Comes First by Ian Kerner.

While targeted to men, this book is a must read for all women. It's a virtual encyclopedia of sexual techniques for pleasing women. Buy one copy for yourself and another one for your man.

Sexopedia by Ann Hooper.

Everything you ever wanted to know about sex, beautifully illustrated.

Appendix B

The 101 Secrets Every Woman Should Know

Read a great tip and can't quite remember where you saw it? Well, here are all 101 secrets listed for your pleasure.

1. *He Likes It When You Get Loud* *1*

2. *Having More Sex Boosts Your Libido* *1*

3. *Porn Can Turn You On Too* *2*

4. *Let Go of Your Past to Heat Up Your Present* *5*

5. *Position Yourself for Pleasure: Try Girl on Top
   (Reverse)* *7*

6. *Men Like Women Who Know What They Want* . . *8*

7. *Clothe Yourself in Confidence* *9*

8. *Don't Sabotage Your Sex Life* *11*

9. *Tantric Sex Will Blow Your Mind* *11*

10. *He'll Love Your Lingerie—Especially If You Show
    It Off Before You Buy It* *14*

11. *He Likes How You Smell Down There* *15*

12. *Have an Affair (with Him)* *16*

13. *Position Yourself for Pleasure: Try the Cross* .18

14. *Learn to Touch Yourself—and Then Teach Your Man Your Moves* *19*

15. *Try Some Kinky, Freaky Sex* *21*

16. *The Way to a Man's Heart (and Other Parts of His Anatomy) Really Is Through His Stomach* . .*23*

17. *Scheduled Sex Can Be Great Sex* *24*

18. *De-Stress for Amazing Sex* *24*

19. *Turn Your Fantasies into Reality* *26*

20. *Buying a Sex Toy Is Not as Scary as You Think* . .*27*

21. *The Kitchen Can Be Kinky Too* *30*

22. *Position Yourself for Pleasure: Give Him a Lap Dance* *31*

23. *Guys Like Girls Who Give Good Head* *32*

24. *Leave the Lights on for Lustful Lovemaking* . .*37*

25. *Have Fun with Fetishes* *38*

26. *Subtlety Can Be Seductive* *40*

27. *Massage Can Be an Aphrodisiac* *42*

28. *Size Does Matter* *44*

29. *Play a Guessing Game* *45*

30. *Your Marriage Is More Important Than Your Kids* *46*

31. *A Trench Coat Is Always in Style* *48*

32. *You Can Get Off Without Letting Him In* . . . *49*

33. *The Female Libido Does Exist* *51*

34. *He Wants You to Want Him* *53*

35. *Position Yourself for Pleasure: Try the Lotus* . *55*

36. *Don't Be Critical* *55*

37. *It's Okay to Do It During That Time of the Month* *57*

38. *Sleep* Au Naturel *59*

39. *Men Love Foreplay, Too* *61*

40. *You Can Learn to Love Oral Sex* *64*

41. *Your Man Will Thank You for Doing Those Kegels* *67*

42. *Knowledge Is Power—Especially When We're Talking about Orgasms* *69*

43. *Intimacy and Desire Go Hand in Hand* *70*

44. *Viagra Isn't the Only Miracle Pill* *72*

45. *Three Can Be Great Company in the Bedroom* 74

46. *Lube Is a Girl's Best Friend* *76*

47. *Sometimes, Kinky Isn't Better* *78*

48. *Position Yourself for Pleasure: Try the Bridge* . . *79*

49. *Anal Sex Can Actually Be Amazing* *80*

50. *Keep It Clean* *83*

51. *Dirty Talk Rocks* *84*

52. *Know What Gets You Hot and Bothered* *86*

53. *He Likes Compliments as Much as You Do* . . . *93*

54. *Phone Sex Works! Give It a Try* *96*

55. *Watch Yourself Do It* *96*

56. *Talk about Your Sex Life* *97*

57. *Condoms Can Be Sexy* *101*

58. *Get Kinky and Try Spanking* *103*

59. *Stop Smoking for Steamier Sex* *106*

60. *Give Your Partner the Ultimate Sexual Experience* *107*

61. *There's More Than One Kind of Orgasm*. *110*

62. *Use Steamy (Instant) Messages to Seduce Your Man* *113*

63. *Turn the Temperature Up — or Down — for Hot Sex*. *114*

64. *Position Yourself for Pleasure: Get Kinky with Girl on Top* *115*

65. *Letting Him Look but Not Touch Is a Total Turn-On* *116*

66. *Contraception Is a Great Wingman* *116*

67. *Sex Toys Can Strengthen Your Orgasm* *121*

68. *Keep the Spark Alive* *123*

69. *Role-Play It Up*. *126*

70. *Experience the Beach in the Buff*. *128*

71. *Go Back to Basics* *129*

72. *Fulfill Your Freaky Fantasies* *133*

73. *Honest Couples Have the Best Sex* *137*

74. *Position Yourself for Pleasure: Try Oral with Manual Stimulation* *137*

75. *Help Him Get Hard* *138*

76. *Have Hot Sex, Even If Your Kids Are Home* . . *142*

77. *Show Some Skin* *143*

78. *Position Yourself for Pleasure: Try the Deep Stick* *144*

79. *Enjoy a Clothing-Optional Weekend* *144*

80. *Get Off More Often* *145*

81. *Lose Your Panties for a Good Time* *147*

82. *Spice Things Up for Long-Term Fun* *147*

83. *Sex Toys Provide Variety* *150*

84. *Don't Step Outside the Box* *156*

85. *Massage His Lingham* *156*

86. *Position Yourself for Pleasure: Try Spooning* . . *158*

87. *Don't Forget to Have Fun* *158*

88. *Know When the "O" Shows Up* *160*

89. *Eat and Drink to Feel Sexy* *161*

90. *Be a Little Uptight* *164*

91. *Get Away from It All* *165*

92. *Tantric Sex Gets You Off Over and Over Again* . *166*

93. *Sufficient Sleep Leads to Hot Sex* *169*

94. *Position Yourself for Pleasure: Do It Doggie Style* *170*

95. *Talk about Your Troubles* *171*

96. *Buy Sex Toys in Secret* *172*

97. *Break a Sweat for Better Sex* *172*

98. *Position Yourself for Pleasure: Try the Modified Missionary* *173*

99. *Safe Makes It Sexy* *173*

100. *Come Again* *177*

101. *Happy, Healthy Women Have the Hottest Sex* *179*

Index

About.com, 187

Adam & Eve, 185

Affairs, 16–18

Aging, 145

AIDS, 174–75

Anal orgasms, 112–13

Anal sex, 22, 80–83, 154

Baths, 65–66, 180

BDSM, 133–37, 155

Beaches, 128–29

Birth control, 102, 177

Blaming, 99, 100

Bondage, 133–35, 155

Boredom, 16–18, 123–26, 158–60

Borg, Sonia, 191

Boundaries, sexual, 21–23, 54–55, 92–93, 128

Breathing, 1, 25, 166–67

Bridge position, 79

Brooke, Melodoy, 188

Bullet vibrators, 152–53

Carlson, Paul, 186

Casual sex, 89

Chalker, Rebecca, 190

Cheating, 16

Children, 46–48, 142–43

Chocolate, 31, 163

Cigarettes, 106–7

Cleanliness, 15–16, 65–66, 83–84

Clitoral orgasms, 110–11

Clitoral Truth, The (Chalker), 190

Clitoral vibrators, 151

Clitoris, 19, 20, 50

Clothing. *See also* Lingerie

confidence and, 9–10

not wearing lingerie, 147

revealing, 143–44

for strip teases, 62

trench coat only, 48–49

turn-ons and, 87

Clothing-optional weekends, 144–45

Communication

about anal sex, 82, 83

about boundaries, 92–93

about dirty talk, 84–85

about fantasies, 22–23, 91

about frequency of sex, 124–25

about oral sex, 34–36, 66

about safe sex, 118

criticism and, 55–57, 71–72

between partners, 54, 72, 97–101, 125–26, 132, 171–72

Compliments, 93–95

Condoms

anal sex and, 81

embarrassment about, 102–3

joint decisions about, 117–18

lubricants and, 77
pre-cum and, 119–20
as sexy, 101–3
STDs and, 118, 120–21, 174,
177
types of, 101–2
Confidence, 8–10, 67, 129,
146–47
Contraception, 102, 116–21,
177. *See also* Condoms
Cooking, 23
Cooper, Amy, 191
Criticism, 55–57, 71–72, 93
Cross position, 18–19
Cuddling, 114–15

Deep Stick position, 144
Dental dams, 174, 175
Desire, 60–61, 70–72. *See also*
Libido
Diet, 161–63, 180
Dildos, 27–30, 153, 154, 170
Dirty talk, 84–85, 96
Discovery Channel, 186
Discreet vibrators, 151–52
Doggie Style position, 170–71
Domination, 135–36
Duration of sex, 122

Eden Fantasys, 185
Egg vibrators, 152–53
EHow, 185

Emails, 17, 113
Embarrassment, 85, 102–3
Emotional baggage, 5–7, 12
Emotional connection, 47, 89,
125–26, 137, 150
Erectile dysfunction, 138–42
Erotica, 2–5
Everything Orgasm Book, The
(Cooper), 191
Exercise, 172–73
Eye contact, 34

Facial expressions, 35
Faking orgasms, 160
Fantasies
acting out, 26–27
BDSM, 133–37
communication with partner
about, 22–23, 91
role-playing, 86–87
women's fantasies about other
women, 74
Fantasy Box, 156
Female ejaculatory orgasms, 179
Female libido, 51–53, 68, 72–73,
124–25
Fetishes, 38–40, 103–5
Finger vibrators, 152
Food, 31, 53, 161–63, 180
Foreplay, 61–64, 129–30
Freaky sex, 21–23, 38–40,
78–79, 103–5, 133–37

Frequency of sex, 1–2, 53, 78, 123, 124–25

Games
    guessing game, 45–46
    role-playing, 17, 86–87, 126–28, 133–36
    talking dirty, 84–85, 96
Ginko biloba, 73
Girl on Top position, 7–8, 115–16
G-Spot
    finding, 168–69, 170
    orgasms, 19, 20, 111–12, 122, 179
    vibrators for, 151
Guessing game, 45–46

Harnesses, 153–54
Harris, Guido, 185
Health, 179–80, 186, 188
HealthCentral, 186
Hepatitis C, 174–75
Herbal supplements, 140
Herpes, 175
HIV, 174–75
Honesty, 98–99, 125–26, 137, 160, 171
Hooper, Ann, 190, 192
Hygiene, 15–16, 83–84

I Love Female Orgasm (Solot and

Miller), 191
Impotence, male, 138–42
Initiating sex, 53–55
Insecurity, 5–7
Instant messaging, 113–14
Intimacy, 70–72, 188

Jealousy, 5–7

Kegel exercises, 67–69, 164–65
Kerner, Ian, 190, 192
Kinky sex, 21–23, 38–40, 78–79, 103–5, 133–37
Kitchen, erotic items in, 30–31
Korean ginseng, 73

Lap dance position, 31–32
Lap dances, 61, 116
Laughter, 85, 95
Libido
    boosting, 53–53, 72–73, 124–25, 140, 147–50, 162
    emotional connection and, 137, 150
    female, 51–53, 68, 72–73, 124–25
    food and, 53, 161–63, 180
    frequency of sex and, 1–2, 53
    loss of, 148–50, 169–70
    male, 51, 68, 124
    stress and, 24–25
Lighting, 37–38, 108

Lingerie
    fantasies and, 27
    popular types of, 41–42
    purchasing, 14–15, 148
    seduction and, 40
    wearing clothing without, 147
Listening, 100–101
Locations, 88
Long-term relationships, 26, 147–50
Lotus position, 55
Lubricants
    anal sex and, 81, 82
    oral sex and, 33, 36–37
    types of, 76–78
    vaginal intercourse and, 130–31
Lying, 98–99, 125

Male libido, 51, 68, 124
Malinak, Joseph and Sarah Elizabeth, 186
Marriage, 46–48
Massage
    erotic, 42–44, 66, 185
    to reduce stress, 26, 180
    tantric, 107–10, 156–58
Masturbation, 19–21, 38, 49–50, 67–68, 176
Meditation, 25
Menstruation, 57–59
Miller, Marshall, 191

Mirrors, 96–97
Modified Missionary positions, 173
Multiple orgasms, 70, 123, 166–69, 177–79
Mutual masturbation, 21

Nicotine, 106–7
Noise during sex, 1
Nudity, 40–42, 59–61, 128–29, 144–45

Odors, vaginal, 15–16
One Hour Orgasm, The (Schwartz), 190, 191
Online resources, 39, 183–88
Oral sex
    learning to enjoy receiving, 64–67
    during menstruation, 59
    position for manual stimulation with, 137–38
    printed resource on, 191
    STDs and, 174, 176
    tips for giving, 32–37
Oral Sex He'll Never Forget (Borg), 191
Orgasms, 49–50
    aging and, 145
    faking, 160
    female ejaculatory, 179
    frequency of, 145–47

Orgasms—*continued*
 Kegel exercises and, 67–69
 multiple, 70, 123, 166–69,
  177–79
 phases of female orgasm,
  69–70
 printed resources on, 190–92
 recognizing, 160–61
 role of clitoris and vagina in,
  19, 20
 sex toys and, 121–23
 simultaneous, 49, 50
 types of, 50, 110–13
Oxytocin, 60

Pain, 90–91
Parents, 46–48, 142–43
Pelvic floor muscles, 67–69
Penis, massage of, 156–58
Penis rings, 154
Penis size, 44–45
Perineum, 157–58
Personas, 86–87
Pheromones, 15
Phone sex, 96–97
Physical activity, 172–73
Pornography, 2–5, 88–89, 124
Positions
 Bridge, 79
 Cross, 18–19
 Deep Stick, 144
 Doggie Style, 170–71

Girl on Top, 7–8, 115–16
 lap dance, 31–32
 Lotus, 55
 Modified Missionary, 173
 for oral sex with manual
  stimulation, 137–38
 spooning, 158
 in vaginal intercourse, 131
 website on, 187
Pre-cum, 119–20
Pregnancy, 58, 119–20
Printed resources, 189–92

Quality time, 52

Relationships
 long-term, 26, 147–50
 preventing boredom in, 16–
  18, 123–26, 158–60
 previous, 5–7
 sexual desire in, 70–72
 website on troubles in, 186
Relaxing
 during anal sex, 82–83
 during oral sex, 65–66
 orgasms and, 146
Remote vibrators, 152
Resources on sexuality
 online, 39, 183–88
 printed, 189–92
Restraints, 90, 92, 155
Reverse Girl on Top position, 7–8

Role-playing, 17, 86–87, 126–28, 133–36

Safe sex, 116–21, 173–77
Scheduled sex, 24
Schwartz, Leah and Bob, 190, 191
Secret meetings, 18
Seduction, 40–42, 48–49
Semen, 118–19, 120
Sex drive. *See* Libido
Sexopedia (Hooper), 190, 192
Sexting, 96, 113
Sex toys
    anal, 154
    buying, 27–30, 172
    dildos, 27–30, 153, 154, 170
    harnesses, 153–54
    homemade, 154–55
    orgasms and, 121–23
    penis rings, 154
    proper care and handling of, 83–84
    restraints and bondage toys, 155
    vaginal intercourse and, 132–33
    vibrators, 27–30, 121–22, 123, 150–53
Sexual boundaries, 21–23, 54–55, 92–93, 128
Sexual confidence, 8–10, 67, 129, 146–47
Sexually transmitted diseases (STDs)
    birth control and, 177
    condoms and, 118, 120–21, 174, 177
    masturbation and, 176
    oral sex and, 174, 176
    types of, 174–75
Sexual peak, 34
Sexual response cycle, 69–70
She Comes First (Kerner), 190, 192
Sheknows.com, 184
Showering with partners, 65–66
Silicone-based lubricants, 77–78, 81
Silverbergy, Cory, 187
Silverman, Maya, 185
Simultaneous orgasms, 49, 50
Sleep, 59–61, 169–70, 180
Smoking, 106–7
Solot, Dorian, 191
Spanking, 103–5
Sperm, 118–19
Spooning position, 158
Spoons, wooden, 30–31
Squirting, 179
St. John's Wort, 73
Stress, 24–26, 180
Stretching, 26

Strip clubs, 63
Strip teases, 61–64, 116
Submission, 136
Subtlety, 40–42
Supplements for libido, 53,
72–73, 140
Tantra, 11–14, 52, 166–69, 184,
187
Tantric massage, 107–10, 156–58
Tara, Carla, 184
Tea, 25
Temperature, 114–15
Text messages, 96, 113
Threesomes, 74–76
Turn-ons, 8–9, 86–93, 116, 168

Vacations, 165–66
Vaginal odors, 15–16
Vaginal orgasms, 19, 20, 110–12,
121–22
Vaginal tightening cream, 164–65
Vaginoplasty, 164
Viagra, 140–41
Vibrance cream, 73
Vibrators, 27–30, 121–22, 123,
150–53

Walking, 25
Water-based lubricants, 77, 81,
130
Websites, 183–88
Withdrawal method, 118
Wooden spoons, 30–31

Yoga, 52

Zestra Feminine Arousal Fluid,
73

About the Authors

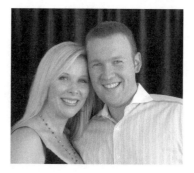

Dan and Jennifer live in Frisco, Texas, and are the founders and senior editors of *www.AskDanAndJennifer.com*, which has been referred to as "The Best & Most Popular Dating, Love, and Sex Advice Column on the Internet Today." AskDanAndJennifer.com has become the premier website about relationships and sexuality on the Internet. The site has achieved a reader base of more than 450,000 readers per month with a strong following from many highly successful authors and bloggers and their content is syndicated on many other popular websites.

In addition, Dan and Jennifer are featured content providers for YouTube, Revver, and Veoh. Their more than 400 videos receive 2–4 million views every month. They provide a refreshing, nonjudgmental, nonbiased approach to relationships and sex. Their beliefs about unconditional love and acceptance are the foundation behind all of their teachings and advice. They have consulted for shows ranging from *Dr. Phil* to *EXTRA* and have been quoted in publications from the *Chicago Sun-Times* to the *Miami Herald*.